THE
CANCER
SOLUTION

A Peltec Publishing Book

Published by Peltec Publishing Co., Inc.
4400 North Federal Hwy., Suite 210
Boca Raton, Florida 33431
Tel. 1 800 214-3645

DEDICATION...

TO MARCIA, MY FRIEND. WIFE AND MOTHER OF MY CHILDREN, WHO WAS MUTILATED AND DESTROYED BY THE FOUR HORSEMAN OF THE NEW APOCALYPSE

* ORTHODOX MEDICINE *

* THE PHARMACEUTICAL INDUSTRY *

* THE FDA AND THE NIH *

* CITIZENS AND INDUSTRIES WHO DESECRATE OUR LIVES AND OUR PLANET *

- SHE DIED OF BRAIN CANCER AFTER UNNECESSARY SURGERY AND HUMILIATING AND NOXIOUS RADIATION.

CONTENTS

Chapter 7

VITAL VITTLES -
VITAMINS AND MINERALS

Chapter 8

WHEN THE PEOPLE FIGHT BACK - VICTORY!

Chapter 12

LET YOUR MEDICINE BE YOUR FOOD

(Items To Use In Your Meals)

Chapter 13
OTHER SIGNIFICANT THERAPIES

Chapter 14
IMMUNE STIMULANTS

Chapter 15

OTHER PRODUCTS TO CONSIDER - MAYBE!

Not so natural, Not so safe.

Chapter 16

THERAPEUTIC PROGRAMS FOR SPECIFIC CANCERS - YOU MIGHT CONSIDER FIRST

Chapter 17

VERY INTERESTING! -

Chapter 18

PARTING THOUGHTS OF A
MEDICAL HERETIC

Chapter 19

A HELPING HAND

*** ALL ITEMS THAT ARE DOUBLE-STARRED (**) ARE, IN THE AUTHORS OPINION, ESSENTIAL TO SUCCESSFUL THERAPY. A SINGLE STAR (*) INDICATES EXTREME USEFULLNESS.

PREFACE

The treatment for cancer throughout the modern and industrial world has been a total disaster and a failure. The cost of treating (killing and mutilating) cancer patients in the USA alone is over a one hundred billion dollars a year. The Wall Street Journal on 22. February, 1991, in an article discussing a new drug called Neupojen, stated that this drug would cost patients between six to ten thousand dollars per year. The incredible irony is that this drug is used to counteract the toxic affects of chemotherapy and therefore is not really in any way directed at the cancer itself. Recently an Office for Unconventional Medical Practices was established within the National Institutes of Health in the United States. Although many will find hope in this new government agency, I remain sceptical. In the 35 years that I had practiced medicine, I had heard many promises but have seen little accomplished.

The "cancer establishment" is a network of extremely powerful and wealthy companies whose members sit on the boards of many non-profit organizations. They literally control and direct all cancer research within the USA and throughout the world. One needs only to read an excellent expose like "The Cancer Industry" by Ralph W. Moss or the "Politics of Cancer" by S.S. Epstein, to get an idea of the influence that the medical-pharmaceutical-chemical complex has over the National Cancer Institute, the American Cancer Society and all the major comprehensive cancer centers. Although these centers are non-profit they simply serve their masters by suppressing most, if not all, non-patentable treatments in favor of the expensive therapies that have wrought havoc with patients while losing the war against cancer. It pours untold billions into the coffers of the "cancer industry". While the incidence of the major cancers has increased, the famous "5-year survival" rate has remained virtually the same.

In recent years a growing number of doctors, nurses and other para-professionals, and even more importantly, the public, have taken increasing notice of natural therapies. They are putting their trust in those doctors who have the foresight and the intelligence to look into methods that have been successful for many centuries. The purpose of this book is to present, in a clear and concise manner, all of the therapies available to those individuals who choose to exercise their freedom of choice by treating and taking care of their own bodies. During the last ten years of my practice, I utilized many therapies that were not in the main stream of medicine. They were safe, non-toxic and very effective.

When I retired, I travelled and researched other therapies available outside of the United States. I spoke with many doctors and patients who were getting excellent results from these alternative therapies and witnessed their successes first-hand. It is time to seriously question and reject the standard orthodox cancer treatments of surgery, radiation and chemotherapy, except in a very few instances when these therapies, with stringent modifications, might be acceptable. It has been frequently argued that these are the only tools of a scientific approach. However, I would argue, that if this is the scientific approach, I can think of better ways to die.

Take notice, that in the presentation of all the "alternative therapies" discussed in this book, I have used references from scientific sources. The major journals rarely contain articles that confirm the usefulness of natural therapies because they rely on advertisements from the powerful pharmaceutical companies. The references that I have used come from the arcane journals that are not frequently read by most doctors. However, the value of a scientific article is not dependent upon the number of doctors that read it.

I strongly advise that when you have read this book and have made a decision to use some of the therapies for your own problem, that you speak to your doctor about it and ask his opinion. If the doctor gives you an opinion, always ask for the source of his information. Too often, doctors simply say "Oh, that doesn't work." or "Which quack did you hear that from?". Ask him very simply, "How do you know it doesn't work?" or "Could you tell me where you read that?" or "How do you know it?" If he doesn't give you resource material and instead repeats a statement similar to what you have heard from the media or from some major organization, then you know that you are just listening to propaganda. It is the same old pseudo-scientific nonsense that has blocked or suppressed some incredibly wonderful therapies in favor of the poisons produced for profit. If your doctor does not have any information about the safer natural therapies, show him the information in this book and all of the references. Many doctors have open minds but are not aware of the fact that a wall of silence has been placed around them.

You may have difficulty in obtaining some of the therapies mentioned in this book. Some of them may be obtained outside of your country. In the USA this is particularly true because the FDA has literally pressured the Congress under the guise of protecting the public to keep time-honored cultural and natural therapies out of the hands of the general public. If you look at the record of the FDA it becomes obvious that they are serving interests other than yours and mine.

The purpose of this book is very simple. I want to discuss all of the therapies and then present a general basic approach to all cancers. I will then list under each type of cancer the specific therapies which can be added to the basic formula. I tried to keep everything clear and concise while at the same time give you the background information and references that are important for you to know. In this way you can make an informed choice when considering their use. Remember, that you can't tell the good guys from the bad guys by the clothes they wear. However, with the information provided in this book you will be able to intelligently question your therapist. Don't be intimidated and remember that a doctor is a teacher. If your physician resents questions from his "student", he is obviously not an educator. If he is not an educator, he is not a doctor.

The majority of the over 1000 references in this book are from the scientific literature. The average doctor relies on two or three journals and a yearly conference to provide him with the information provided in the over ten thousand journals published. He or she is therefore deprived of the opportunity to know what is really out there. In addition, knowledge from other schools of thought and practice is condemned as "quackery" and therefore believed to be heresy. In recent years the experience of thousands of years surfaces as a "new" finding. It appears as though modern cancer research is finally rediscovering the past in spite of the suppressive efforts of the FDA, the AMA and the Pharmaceutical Industry. The public and many physicians, however, cannot wait for them to learn the basics they should have learned in school. The therapies presented in this book are almost entirely non-toxic, with a few exceptions that may be mildly toxic. They offer a distinct advantage over anything that orthodox medicine has to present. I argue this point of view in various sections of the book, the ultimate choice as to what you do will be yours.

J. Period Cearns, in his article in the Scientific American of November 1985, points very clearly to the fact that the war against cancer has not made any significant advances in cure rates for many decades. The protestations of the establishment hold little credence when they declare that their approach is the "only way". In 1987 the U.S. Court of Appeals in Schneider versus Revici, clearly stated that it is your constitutional right to seek a treatment of your choice. The massive medical centers are impressive monuments to modern technology. They excel in diagnostic ability. But once having accomplished that goal, these great edifices become tombs for the medically maimed. With great authority and pomposity, they assume a deified presence and solemnly direct the course of your life on a hopeless path towards death. You sign legal documents absolving them of their arrogant ignorance and intended crimes. Your questions are taken as affront to their lofty position and an insult to their supreme intelligence, for they truly believe that no other answer exists but what they have to offer. They brand as heretics and venomously denounce their own colleagues who have dared question their rituals. They excommunicate those who seek a rational and non-destructive path to salvation. My advice - find physicians with open minds and the courage of their convictions. **THE ANSWERS YOU SEEK SHOULD NOT BE A DOCTOR'S OPINION BASED ON ANOTHER OPINION. IT SHOULD BE AN OPINION BASED ON CLINICAL EXPERIENCE, OBSERVATION AND ACTUAL FACT.**

Chapter 1

From Victim To Victor - Understanding The Problem

YOUR PASSPORT TO LIFE

Welcome, I am so glad that you have decided to fight cancer, rather than succumb to this terrible disease. More importantly, I am glad that you selected this book to educate yourself, so that you can successfully exercise your right to informed consent, with knowledge that would not ordinarily be made available to you. This book will provide you with information, much of which has been known for centuries and even millennia.

Virtually all of the therapies presented in this book are backed by a substantial number of scientific articles, have been used with a reasonable degree of success and are safe to use.

In keeping with the doctrine of informed consent and in view of the fact that there are a large number of individuals who are sceptical about the accepted modalities of chemotherapy, surgery and radiation., it is the sole purpose of this book to present all of the therapies proven and unproven that have gained at least some appreciable success in various parts of the world.

It is strongly advised that you confer with a competent practitioner in matters dealing with the treatment of disease! It is intended to enable you to intelligently exercise your informed freedom of choice!

It is knowledge that will enable you to better deal with the many daily challenges to your health. This is a book about methods of healing that may differ from the consensus of opinion held by members of the medical profession, although no **actual** consensus opinion has ever been taken or established. It is about therapies that physicians do not learn about in medical school, despite the fact that physicians have used them for ages. It is about healthy living that even Hippocrates recommended. It is about therapies that many physicians would like to use, but dare not, out of fear that they would be accused of practicing with methods not generally accepted by the medical community in which they live and work.

The information you will read in this book is not available to you from the average "establishment" health practitioner. These sincere physicians, though seriously limited in basic therapeutic knowledge that was a part of the medical armamentarium for centuries, are often referred to as practitioners of "orthodox " medicine. In fact, they are not practicing orthodox medicine. They are practicing current establishment medicine.

THE BIRTH OF PSEUDO - SCIENCE

With the beginnings of the pharmaceutical industry and the introduction of " drugs", many doctors discarded the knowledge they had gained over thousands of years. In the quest for the chemical magic potions or "bullets" that would destroy disease, they abandoned the use of diet, herbs, homeopathic remedies, colonic irrigation and other safe (not necessarily by government opinion) and more natural techniques which had survived the test of time. They actively isolated and effectively eliminated those who sought to continue the use of these methods. You wouldn't think, that after the now famous and discredited attacks on such giants as Semmelweis, Pasteur, Freud and hundreds of other great discoverers and contributors to medical knowledge, that the medical community could still be mired in the mud of "consensus medicine" - medicine by vote. It is difficult to believe today that washing one's hands prior to surgery or delivering a baby, was a radical idea, and not in keeping with the mainstream of medicine, just a little over one hundred years ago!

Unfortunately, physicians still belie their claim to being scientists. They cling to the erroneous belief that they are practicing pure science with their narrowly focused double-blind studies. At the same time they ignore that the life process is an extreme complexity of interactions between an organism and its environment, evolving through a slow, prolonged process of adaptation. It is a process that involves the organism itself and the substances upon which it depends for survival. What we call "nature" is all that is, all that has adapted, all that has survived. Anything else is not natural and therefore alien. That which is alien to nature cannot possibly correct what it undoubtedly caused.

Replacing but a part, can never reconstruct the whole, which is assuredly more than the sum of its parts. Maintaining natural relationships in life is both the prevention and the cure.

HIPOCRASY, NOT HIPPOCRATES

Physicians today, are required to practice within the "standards of the community". This does not mean what it seems say. The word "standards" no longer refers to the qualities of high or low, excellent or poor. It now means that you do what everybody else is doing, even though no vote on the matter has been taken. Usually, just one physician is brought in as a witness. He is asked if the treatment in question meets the standard of practice in the community. If he answers no, or that he has never heard of it, then it is not acceptable. These hearings rarely meet the legal requirements of a court of law and any physician that attempts to fight the system, soon finds himself drained of his assets in a futile attempt to find justice. It means that a physician can no longer afford to think creatively and only at great risk would dare to use a thoroughly legal substance to treat a problem, unless a majority of physicians were using it. This completely unscientific attitude of a "closed-mind" exists only at the discretion of the public will. The Supreme Court of the United States has declared that a physician has the right to use a legal medication for any purpose for which he believes it might be effective. However, the State medical associations, through the power of the departments of professional regulation, use "administrative" law to circumvent the courts of law and deprive the citizens of that state, who practice a profession, of their constitutional rights. Unfortunately, in this dictatorship of allopathic medicine and the pharmaceutical industry, it is the patient that ultimately loses.

The very nature of the medical profession, under the influence and deception of the pharmaceutical industry, is one of conflict of interest. True disease prevention, other than the questionable practice of vaccination, is either rejected, too time consuming and in conflict with economic gain. Traditional natural nutritional concepts are therefore a total enigma to most physicians. It is certainly more profitable to dispense with the patient quickly and at a substantial fee, and simply write a prescription regardless of the risks involved to the patients. Everything is ruled by "consensus" and therefore is the "best that is available". It goes unchallenged, because all opposition is unorthodox, unprofessional and "not in keeping with community standards", and therefore illegal and quackery.

The so-called "side effects" of drugs are, in truth, unwanted direct effects. The cumulative result of many of these therapies on the suppression of the immune system, coupled with the multiple insults visited daily upon us from the pollution of our air, food and water, has unquestionably been the reason that the rate of cancer has doubled in the past twenty years. The crime is compounded by establishment medicine's symptomatic approach which leaves the causative factors in tact.

The true orthodox physician, if one uses Hippocrates as the standard, is now referred to as the "alternative" or "wholistic" physician. However, the current common usage exists because establishment allopathic medicine through the efforts of the AMA, which represents less than half the physician population, has successfully gained control of the institutions of learning and the journals that disseminate medical information. They effectively dictate medical consensus. For the most part, there is no conscious conspiracy going on. The physician of today is merely the product of over a century of conditioning in the "legitimate drug" culture. The formative years of modern medicine has left a profound impact on the adult it has grown to be.

The neuroses of arrogance and dogma have made medicine self-destructive and have severely impaired its capacity for creative, or dissident thinking. It has always been the dissident thinker which caused the art and the science of medicine to advance and flourish. Like most neurotics, medicine refuses to believe or is not aware that its behavior is destructive. Therefore, like many neurotics, it will resort to extreme (psychotic) behavior in defense of its position. Sadly, the medical community is not able to see this deficiency in themselves. They simply believe they know it all, or at best they don't believe anyone else knows more. The Physician may observe a response occurring repeatedly in the care of many patients, but until it is proven by the "double-blind" method of testing it cannot be accepted as "official". This is unlikely to happen unless the therapy is patentable, otherwise the cost of proving it is prohibitive.

THE MODERN INQUISITION

It is historical fact that the pharmaceutical industry (the oil and chemical industry) has been the major force responsible for the narrow, arrogant and simple-minded path that has brought physicians success in less than ten percent of the diseases they are called upon to treat. The pharmaceutical complex provides research grants, contracts and the advertising support responsible for the existence of the many thousands of journals published each year. This guarantees virtual control over scientific and medical direction and thought. The result has been highly profitable. By creating a dogmatic religious zeal in the search for the "holy Grail", the cure of all disease by drugs, the average physician has become totally intolerant of all other schools of thought and practice. The great majority of physicians are honest, dedicated and sincere scientists. They truly believe that they are on the "cutting edge" of medicine and that anyone that pursues another path is either misguided, ill-informed, a charlatan or a "quack". The modern day inquisitions which take the form of administrative hearings, deny victims of their constitutional rights. They have resulted in the loss of licence to practice medicine and heavy fines for many physicians searching for safer and better ways to treat disease. A period of probation is always added to insure that the victim repents and does not revert to the use of heretical measures in the treatment of patients. There are many thousands of physicians who practice what they believe to be a better brand of medicine, but have to do so in constant fear of discovery. There would be hundreds of thousands more if they were ever given the chance to learn of the non-toxic and effective (by historical usage) therapies available. I mourn for Hippocrates, whose admonitions to **"Above all, do no harm"** and **"Let your food be your medicine and your medicine be your food",** have been discarded in favor of the of the doctrine of the "lesser of the evils". As long as physicians pursue the "magic bullet" and ignore the lessons of thousands of years of knowledge and experience, iatrogenic (medically caused) illness and death will become more prevalent than ever.

The Food and Drug Administration is continuously adding, eliminating or revising information on the use of medicines, because of serious problems noted long after the FDA cleared them for safety and effectiveness. In spite of the fact that they were born of the "double-blind" birth process, these changes interestingly enough were discovered, not by double-blind techniques, but by anecdotal evidence. The actual occurrence of the cover-up and masking of the failures in the "infallability" of the double-blind criteria of proof is much greater than admitted or known because of the limitations inherent in the allopathic philosophy and its intolerance to any other point of view. As long as the dictatorship of allopathic medicine reigns, fostered by the powerful and politically influential pharmaceutical industry, the public will be denied the right of informed freedom of choice in health and disease care.

THE DOUBLE-EDGE SWORD

Modern medicine has excelled in advancing the technology for diagnosis and in the treatment of crisis situations. Surgical procedures have been developed that accomplish miraculous results and have not only saved many lives, they have brought or restored a decent quality of life to millions. When analyzed carefully, these advances have been mechanical in character, but still ultimately rely on the natural healing processes for success. Sadly, these technological miracles have, in many in stances, been abused out of ignorance and the lust for profit. It is in the area of crisis medicine that physicians can boast of most of their achievements. Yet, it represents only a pitifully small part of the problems it faces. Lest undue credit be sought for antibiotics and vaccines, it should be pointed out that the great advances in sanitation and hygiene have been far more responsible for the control of infectious disease. In these instances, only those methods which utilize natural means are ultimately safe and effective.

The incredible gains in the interest of public health in the area of hygiene and sanitation are now being overshadowed and lost. A new disaster has been in the making and is being caused by the same industrial revolution that brought us the technologies of improved sanitation. Like the surgeon's knife, most scientific, medical and technological advances have proven to be a double-edged sword. We learn daily that some drug, chemical, pesticide or food additive is being removed from the marketplace or is under serious suspicion after many years of use. We now know, without any doubt, that millions more are dying from the "advances" of modern medicine and science than from all the forces of nature and mankind's war machines combined. The reasons for this will be clearly explained in chapter 2 " The Scourge Of Mankind Or Mankind's Scourge?"

HOW HERESY IS BORN

It seems appropriate at this point to explain how I became a heretic to "establishment" medicine and rediscovered the true roots of the real "orthodox" medicine. For more than twenty years I practiced establishment medicine. I truly believed and was extremely proud that I was amongst the elite of the healing arts, the real physician, the true physician - I was an "M.D."! If you had asked me fifteen years ago what I thought about the other healers, I would have, in no uncertain words, attacked them as practicing unscientific witchcraft. My salvation as a true physician, unbeknownst to me, began very early in my career. I yearned for better answers and instinctively was attracted to anything new and different as long as it did no harm. It would take me many years however, before I was to question the benefit of the basic allopathic philosophy and the methods in which I had been trained.

I learned hypnosis in 1958, the year it was accepted by the AMA. In 1960, by fortuitous circumstance, I started to use "trigger point" injections as described in a well-known medical journal by Janet Travell, M.D. (President Kennedy's physician). For eleven years I used this technique very successfully in the management of pain syndromes. When Nixon visited China, the periodicals carried stories of a reporter who had an appendectomy under acupuncture anesthesia. The now familiar acupuncture charts were often reproduced in the newspaper and magazine articles. I became suspicious and compared the "trigger points" to acupuncture points - they were identical! I had been doing acupuncture by injection (often injecting just vitamins into the points) for eleven years without knowing it.

In 1963, I was introduced to Carlos Lamar, M.D., one of the early pioneers in chelation therapy (more about this incredible modality later). In spite of astounding and miraculous results, I was frightened away from continuing its use by an article which appeared in a major medical journal claiming chelation as the cause of death in two patients. A careful analysis of the article would have revealed this conclusion as totally invalid. I was too young and naive at the time to ever question one of the bibles of establishment medicine. Chelation is unquestionably the best solution to coronary atherosclerotic disease. It is without a doubt preferable to by-pass surgery which does not prolong life and kills six percent of the patients (see chapter on chelation). I often think of the many lives I could have saved and the improved quality of life I could have afforded my patients had I been wiser and more experienced. Today, chelation is legal in many states. In the State of Florida, the Supreme Court ruled that it can be used for purposes other than mercury or lead poisoning. Yet, in Florida, a physician can lose his license if he recommends its use in place of the deadly and 90% useless by-pass surgery - because it is not the "standard" of practice of the community. In Florida, one physician who tested the use of two foods in a diet program, had his license suspended for one year because his study, which was double-blinded, indicated they were effective. The State said they were therefore "drugs" if they were effective!

My appetite to find other methods grew, but still I never questioned the methods of establishment medicine. My practice however, consisted mostly of the management of chronic pain problems without drugs. Although I did not spend much of my time treating other illnesses, I gradually held back on using as many medicines as my colleagues did for most problems. My patients seemed to do as well and often times much better than with the orthodox approach. Fortunately, the medicare program has curtailed the excessive use of many medications.

Then in 1978, my wife developed cancer of the brain. I dutifully concurred with the recommended and accepted therapies of surgery and radiation. This exceptionally beautiful and brilliant psychotherapist, wife and mother, was reduced to inhuman status by the insanity of modern medicine. She died twenty-one months later. The "state-of-the-art" therapy for cancer had achieved its usual results - degradation, debilitation, loss of dignity, loss of quality of life, big fees and the holy proclamation "the best that could be done, had been done". Some of our most respected scientists and even our government have questioned many tests and therapies and in fact refuse reimbursement for them. In cancer, many, questionably effective therapies, remain in use simply because they are all that is available. **SAFE ALTERNATIVES ARE ALWAYS REJECTED!**

CHOICES

Life is a series of choices. I am sure everyone has asked themselves, "What would my life be like if I had ... " and then finished the sentence with any one of the countless pivotal decisions they could have made along the path of life. There is a basic truth; the decisions we make, are almost always, the only decisions we could have made. This becomes obvious if we simply go back in time and review that particular moment and understand what our feelings, circumstances and knowledge was at that given instant. My life experiences in medicine led

9

me gradually on a path from "establishment" or "orthodox" medicine to what is commonly referred to as "alternative" therapies in the treatment of the ninety percent of the diseases that confront the average physician., the diseases for which the physician has no satisfactory solution. The events of my life, guided by experience, knowledge and circumstance, brought me to the inevitable "place" I occupy today.

Most physicians find it difficult to believe that practitioners outside the mainstream of medicine could accomplish with herbs, diet, homeopathics and change in life-style what they cannot do with drugs (with all their many troubling side-effects). "How," they ask incredulously, "could these crazy doctors come up with a better answer than the great pharmaceutical companies like Merck, Sharp and Dome, Pfizer or Wyeth, with their hand-picked scientists and the hundreds of millions of dollars they spend each year in research?" "How can these doctors know more than the brilliant minds in the finest medical universities in the world?" "Don't you think," they persist in a mocking tone, "that the major pharmaceutical companies would pay millions for the rights to the cure for cancer?" "Do you honestly believe that the officials of our government, many of whom have children, mates or parents dying of cancer, would stand in the way of a cure?" They only ask these questions because they have the arrogance and the ignorance to believe that they can improve on nature. Except in the small percentage of emergent conditions where dramatic artificial measures are required, and here I give them accolades, the belief that they are doing any good at all, is pure myth!

After twenty years of searching and a willingness to learn - after twenty years of experiencing what it was like to have cancer myself and losing my most precious friend, the mother of my children, to cancer - I have found many of the answers. Most importantly, I learned that answers were to be found in the five-thousand year-old, world-wide history of medicine. I learned that old was not necessarily bad and new was not necessarily good. After all, natural "alternative" medicine was based on these many years of experience and much of it taught by the "father of medicine", Hippocrates.

Establishment medicine, at the encouragement, indeed bribery, of the young and brazen upstart pharmaceutical industry, cast aside all previous therapeutics as unscientific and not worthy of consideration. The window to the abundantly rich past was closed, thus dimming the light on future discovery. Interestingly, the most significant successes of the pharmaceutical world, the discovery of antibiotics and insulin, are both obtained from natural substances.

OF CAUSES AND CURES

Throughout history great plagues and epidemics have taken the lives of millions. However, many individuals survived. Why? The answer is obvious. The survivors were those whose immune systems were functioning effectively. The next question, of course, is what adversely effected those who succumbed to the illnesses. The answers, in the context of modern immunological knowledge have been known for more than fifty years. Certainly genetics play an important, but minor role. However, malnutrition, drugs, pollution, radiation of all types, chemicals, steroids and stress and the extremely common and dangerous processing of foods, either individually or in combination, are all major causes. The immune system of the body is primarily composed of the blood and lymph system. However, in reality, it involves a balanced functioning of every system and structure, including every single cell in the body.

The approach of establishment medicine has been to find the "magic bullet" for each disease. This has not and will not likely happen - it is doomed to fail except in a few isolated and rare conditions. The cause of disease is not a single agent with a singular effect. It cannot be stopped even by a "magic bullet". It is pure illusion - a myth! In the majority of medical problems, cancer and all the chronic degenerative diseases, the treatment is often worse than the disease, usually only symptomatic and the consequences horrendous. Until establishment medicine understands that the only intelligent and ultimately successful approach is, first and foremost, prevention, failure will prevail. Secondly, the repair and support of our immune system with natural remedies that do not interfere with normal processes is the best rational and scientific approach. If this is not understood, then the cure for cancer and degenerative diseases will remain, for them, unattainable.

As long as the establishment commits the basic mistake of corrupting bio-chemistry (life-chemistry), it will continue to administer deceptive and ultimately destructive unnatural compounds into the incredibly complex and sensitive biochemistry of the body. Even the synthetic, exact duplicates of what is described as the "active" ingredient of natural herbs, moulds, hormones or enzymes are often, in practical application, not as effective as the original and usually is accompanied by dangerous side-effects. The reason for this is self-evident. A specific compound isolated from its natural environment in the structure of a plant, for example, may lose some synergistic, buffering or even antagonistic action or balance that is present when ingested in its natural form. Although the pharmaceutical companies usually claim that the artificially created product provides a more dependable consistency, better control of the dose and other, sometimes questionable, claims, it is rarely the real truth. The ability to obtain a patent is always the prime concern.

In the spirit of human rights, this book endeavors to pierce the walls of silence that bar access to knowledge about the existence and the efficacy of all the non-toxic therapies available. Many can be still easily obtained in the United States, but they may soon be obscured from public availability by FDA censorship under the guise that the therapeutic claims have not been proven. Other safe and effective therapies, though not proven, can only be obtained by citizens of the U.S.A. by traveling out of the country. This will continue as long as freedom of informed choice in medical care is denied. If the accessibility and equal reimbursement for advanced (natural) therapies are denied, our national debt will continue to rise with nothing to show for it except the highest medical bill in the world. The ineffective and destructive treatments for cancer will continue to maim and dehumanize us, while the incidence of these diseases will increase and we will continue to rank seventeenth or worse in health amongst the nations of the world. It is for this reason that we cite the ultimate deceptions practiced by the Medical-Pharmaceutical-Government complex. It can only be halted by public outcry and it is my hope that you will voice your anger and indignation at this public rape.

ADVANCED IDEAS - "AS OLD AS THE HILLS"

If ever you are faced with the terribly frightening diagnosis of cancer or any other chronic incapacitating or deadly disease, do not rely solely on the information provided in this book. Gather more information from representatives of several healing philosophies. Ask of all of them, especially those of establishment medicine;

1. **How long do you estimate I have if I follow all your advice? (approximate)**
2. **How long do I have if I do nothing at all? (approximate)**
3. **What are all the side effects?**
    - AND GET IT IN WRITING!

Lastly, I wish to stress that prevention of all disease can be accomplished mostly by the way we as individuals conduct our daily lives, and if we succeed in our insistence that the government increases restrictions on the pollution of our land, air and water and eliminate the harmful and destructive processing of foods. The treatment of existing disease, however, is another matter and does require the guidance and assistance of a trained professional. **Do not be fooled by anyone who claims a cure for any disease with just one therapy.** It is unlikely that a singular substance or device will result in a cure or effective prevention. Put simply, **"You cannot bake a cake with flour alone!"**. We have adapted to our environment over millions of years, but the incredible changes in the past century have been too many and too quick for adaptation to take place. It is necessary to take a comprehensive approach in order to succeed in repairing the body's defenses and in providing adequate protection against recurrences. This can be accomplished by using what I call the **Biological Immuno-Regeneration** concept of healing, a program encompassing the five major ingredients necessary if the successful elimination of disease is to become a reality. They are easily recalled by using the acronym - **I.D.E.A.S.!**™

> **I**mmune support
> **D**iet fortification
> **E**nergy enhancement
> **A**nti-pathogenic (non-toxic measures)
> **S**pirit, Mind and Body

I believe that this is "advanced medicine", it follows a strict Hippocratic approach. It abides by the pledge to, "Above all, do no harm." The treatment must be non-toxic and the cornerstone of any effective therapy must be a change in life-style, diet and the quality of the food ingested. It has become increasingly evident that organic foods, those grown without artificial fertilizers, pesticides and not exposed to chemicals, excessive heating, gassing or irradiation, are the safest and most nourishing foods for your health. Many of these processes have been permitted without adequate testing or confirmation of their safety.

Others have remained on the shelf in spite of abundant evidence that they are harmful and, in the case of processing even condemned by major international organizations. The discontinuance of at least some products by the FDA is further evidence of this fact.

Take careful note of the paragraph that follows and the words which I have emphasized. It illustrates a truth that was understood more than two thousand years ago, yet only recently acknowledged, in part, by establishment medicine.

" *WHEREFORE I SAY THAT SUCH CONSTITUTIONS AS SUFFER QUICKLY AND STRONGLY FROM **ERRORS IN DIET** ARE WEAKER THAN OTHERS THAT DO NOT;*
(a poor diet lowers resistance to disease)
AND THAT A WEAK PERSON IS IN A STATE VERY NEARLY APPROACHING TO ONE IN DISEASE....
AND THIS I KNOW, MOREOVER, THAT TO THE HUMAN BODY IT MAKES A GREAT DIFFERENCE WHETHER THE BREAD BE FINE OR COARSE, OF WHEAT WITH OR WITHOUT THE HULL, WHETHER MIXED WITH MUCH OR WITH LITTLE WATER, STRONGLY WROUGHT OR SCARCELY AT ALL, BAKED OR RAW....
(processing of food effects your health)
WHOEVER PAYS NO ATTENTION TO THESE THINGS, OR PAYING ATTENTION, DOES NOT COMPREHEND THEM, HOW CAN HE UNDERSTAND THE DISEASES WHICH BEFALL A MAN:
(if you don't know about nutrition, don't call yourself a doctor!)
FOR BY EVERY ONE OF THESE THINGS, A MAN IS

AFFECTED AND CHANGED THIS WAY OR THAT, AND THE WHOLE OF HIS LIFE IS SUBJECTED TO THEM, WHETHER IN HEALTH, CONVALESCENCE OR DISEASE. *NOTHING ELSE, THEN, CAN BE MORE IMPORTANT OR MORE NECESSARY TO KNOW THAN THESE THINGS. "*

HIPPOCRATES 400 B.C.
****

SPECIAL NOTICE - THE OBVIOUS!

The law states that you should be informed that this book is not intended to give you medical advice about your specific problem, as well it should not. First of all, you and I have never met. Secondly, I am not your doctor and I haven't examined you or reviewed your case. However, free speech and the dissemination of knowledge, though in grave danger, are still permitted. It is in this spirit, and with great respect and belief that the individual is the final arbiter in their live's decisions, that I offer other options as possible alternative methods to consider in the treatment of disease - especially cancer. I will only provide you with the knowledge, but the choice, my friend, is yours!

TRUTH AND UNDERSTANDING - THE WAY TO GO!

I am happy and grateful to have this opportunity to offer you information that I know will more likely help you achieve optimal health and a happier and more rewarding life than allopathic medicine can. I am sure that reading this book will be an enriching, educational and healing experience, signaling a new beginning filled with hope. My life as a physician has convinced me that it will be **"Your Passport To Life"**. It will give you the knowledge necessary to assist you in becoming a successful partner with your physician in your journey out of disease and into a joyful and healthy life. Because it is an adventure in living and learning, it is preferable that you think of yourself as a partner, rather than a patient in the medical relationship. Learn from each other and communicate with honesty and understanding. This is the surest way for you to achieve your desired goal.

It is important that you understand that the therapies and concepts you will read about have in some instances, been reported successful in the treatment of millions of patients. Though the modalities discussed have not been subjected to double-blind testing, remember that neither has more than 80% of the therapies used in allopathic medicine (1978 - investigation by The Office of Technological Assessment, at the direction of the U.S. Congress). The cost of double-blind testing is estimated to now be in the hundreds of millions of dollars and is out of the question unless the method is patentable and the investment therefore recoverable. This is the reason the pharmaceutical industry has pushed for such expensive requirements. This may seem contradictory, but it is not. It is an extremely effective way of eliminating competition from hundreds of smaller companies. Why not spend hundreds of millions in order to make billions! It is not, as some might have you believe, only an interest in safety, efficacy and the public good. The extreme power of the FDA, though at first fought by the pharmaceutical industry is now welcomed by the giant corporations as the best means of eliminating competition ever devised. Their influence over the FDA still remains and is obvious. Why else would a health supplement like L-tryptophan be removed from the shelves permanently because of a contaminated batch from Japan, while countless contaminated drugs have been simply recalled and then been allowed to be replaced. An amateur biochemist knows that an <u>essential</u> amino acid cannot be dangerous, especially one that is found in abundance in such foods as milk and fish. Could it be that L-tryptophan was safely replacing sleeping pills and tranquilizers without any of the side-effects and danger of addiction? Or was it because they were much cheaper and didn't require a trip to the physicians office for a prescription?

A PERSONAL NOTE

I am a bladder cancer survivor for more than twenty years. The tumor was snipped out surgically - but why didn't it recur as most bladder cancers do? In my medical opinion the major reasons I have survived are these:
1. I have virtually eliminated artificial chemicals, fried foods and excessive protein, fats, sugar (plus refined carbohydrates) and processed foods from my diet. It actually began with the elimination of saccharin which had just been announced to have been linked with **bladder cancer!**
2. I have vowed not to let things grind me down (minimizing stress).
3. I have learned to live in the moment.

4. I have stopped taking medicines of any type except when they are absolutely necessary (extremely rare circumstances).

5. I take supplements to counter the effects of the pollution in our air, food and water. This includes certain foods, like relatively fresh cold-pressed linseed oil, which can be difficult to obtain in their natural state.

6. I take chelation (though not as regularly as I should - monthly).

7. I periodically use ozone intravenously. The FDA has condemned its use, even though when used properly it is safe, legal, and is utilized by thousands of physicians throughout the world and its value in medicine goes back more than one hundred years (Dade County Medical Journal - **1885** and hundreds of medical articles published by the Proceedings of the International Ozone Medical Association).

Healing is a time of hope and learning to live in the moment. Take my hand, now is the time live, now is the time to heal, now is the time to learn!
"THE POWER OF THE HUMAN SPIRIT OVER ADVERSITY IS WITHOUT LIMIT"

****

Chapter 2

The Scourge Of Mankind, Or Mankind's Scourge?

CANCER!

Cancer is no longer a mysterious disease. However, the establishment still presents that image. The means by which the prevention of cancer can be achieved is obvious, but orthodoxy has only conceded one of these methods while still pretending that the causes of cancer are still unknown. In 1989, The American Cancer Society finally proclaimed that we could prevent 35% of all cancers with diet alone. The causes of most cancers are known, and it is far easier to prevent them than it is to cure them. The purpose of this book is to do just that, provide you with information on which you can better choose a path to ultimate health.

There are many simple non-toxic effective treatments for cancer. The cost of proving them has been made impossible by the collusion between the FDA and the pharmaceutical industry. The establishment has deliberately used every imaginable and shameful tactic, some of which are even "strong-arm", to discredit, conceal and destroy these therapies. The reasons are clear. The pharmaceutical industry, which profits in the countless billions from their infamous chemotherapy and all the drugs that usually have to be taken with it to deal with the horrible "side-effects", would lose an enormous income if the truth were known. The medical profession perpetuates the myth for several reasons:

Because medical education and research is largely financed and controlled by the pharmaceutical industry, either directly or indirectly through their political influence, the majority of physicians truly believe in the "magic bullet" that will "someday" be discovered. This attitude took firm hold with the discovery of antibiotics and the legacy of the successful germ theory. Undue credit was bestowed on antibiotics and the dramatic effect of improved sanitation was largely ignored. The fact that the coincidental improvement in hygiene played a far more important role has been generally concealed. Physicians are so indoctrinated in the concept of "better living through chemistry", that they readily believe that natural solutions must be "quackery". Unfortunately there are scoundrel business and scientific entrepreneurs who have given and continue to lend credence to that perception. Doctors truly believe that they have a monopoly on "state of the art" weapons at their disposal, and that all other approaches are the products of ignorance or downright fraud. This inbred arrogance and ignorance has hindered the advance of good medical practice more than any other factor - **I know, I once believed in the same myth.**

The second reason lies in the economic comforts and privilege that this allopathic medical monopoly provides. The Physician has enjoyed a unique status of wealth, power and prestige, unchallenged until recent years. The public is becoming educated and medicine has failed to deliver on one promise after another. Having spent close to forty years in medicine, I know that there are very few physicians who perpetuate the myth knowingly. The rewards tend to dull one's ability to be critical. It is also very difficult to challenge or search for the flaws in the basic meaning of an entire life's work. Can you imagine looking back and having to say to yourself, "I did it all wrong!" ?

Lastly, we have a corrupt, self-serving and often inept government bureaucracy that protects these special powerful interests. They can be vicious and fanatic in their zealousness. The result; pain and suffering, needless deaths and a waste of resources beyond imagination, which has been the greatest single contributing factor responsible for the huge national debt threatening to cripple our nation.

THE CAUSES OF CANCER

In the strictest sense, cancer is not caused by an immune deficiency. Anything, however, alone or in combination with other factors that adversely effect that system and/or any other tissue of the body, thus causing changes in the metabolic processes, can result in a growth pattern that breaks free from the normal genetic code. It will also hinder the ability of protective mechanisms to defend the body. Simply stated, the symbiotic peaceful co-existence developed over many millennia, when disrupted, results in disease or death. Because survival arises from, and depends upon the ability to adapt to the environment, reason tells us that the means for our survival is derived from that environment. The fact that there are populations which do not have a particular type of cancer, or any cancer at all, is tacit evidence that prevention is inherent in life-style, diet, many environmental factors, and in some instances, the fact that "modern medicine" is not available and therefore not one of the causes.

Orthodox medicine has become so dogmatic and confined in its demand for double-blind studies, that it rejects effective applied techniques and remedies that have been used for centuries. The vital role of psycho-neuro-immunological factors have been belittled and relegated disparagingly to what the establishment considers the waste basket of the "placebo". The thinking physician and scientist should be cognizant that any factor in the equations of survival that can be responsible for influencing the outcome of an experiment by as much as fifty-percent, is indeed a major force and not merely a "variable" that can conveniently be excluded. Cancer occurs when a cell's metabolism is effected by chemicals and pharmaceuticals. Prime examples are amyl nitrite ("poppers") causing Kaposi's Sarcoma and saccharine causing bladder cancer. Radiation is a well recognized cause of many types of tumors. It must be remembered here that severe stress can alter the effect of even the body's chemicals on its own tissue. The common denominator, however, depends on whether the body's defenses are functioning well enough to deal with the onslaught and the aberrations by neutralizing their destructive effects. A similar situation exists in relation to infectious agents and the myriad of causes of degenerative disease. Any therapy that attacks the immune system, poisons or disrupts the cell structure or function, cannot be legitimately considered for use. The time supposedly "gained" is too often inconsequential and the effects of the therapy is almost always brutal and dehumanizing. The quality of life can scarcely be called anything more than a "living death". If the cause of disease, including cancer, is an inadequate defense or an indefensible attacker, which it assuredly is, then destroying the defenses of the body therapeutically, guaranties a fatal outcome. This is the insanity of "hi-tech, state-of-the-art, modern medicine". The Merck Manual, the "physicians bible", has since its first edition in 1952, listed all of the causes of immune deficiency. Thousands of articles have appeared in scientific journals throughout the world citing the many specific causes of cancer. The elimination of these dread diseases is possible today. Commitment to a sane approach is all that is needed.

****

HEREDITARY FACTORS

It has been estimated that only about **5% of all cancers are due to hereditary factors.** Melanoma and cancers in children primarily fall into this category. A. G. Knudson of the Fox Chase Cancer Center in Philadelphia, Pennsylvania, relates that distortions of certain chromosomes in our genetic structure, appear to be responsible for different types of tumors. Notably, **chromosome 13 is involved in retinoblastoma of the eye** and **chromosome 8 in Wilms' Tumor.** There is a greater risk of developing cancer at some time in your life if your blood is type **A or AB.** Don't let it worry you, simply lower the risk by eliminating all the other factors. The fact that **malignant melanoma** seems to run in families should alert family members to appearance of any unusual discolored lesions of the skin. If there is, in fact, a particular type of cancer that has shown up for several generations, this too, should act as a cautionary sign and prompt extra vigilance for the occurrence of that type of tumor in other family members.

RATIONAL EFFECTIVE THERAPY

Dr. Otto Warburg won the Nobel Prize in science in 1931 for demonstrating that a cancer cell had the metabolism of a plant cell. He described the process succinctly as "fermentation". This meant that the metabolic process was the opposite to that of normal tissues which are composed of animal cells. This gives us the most important clue to follow in developing a successful approach to the prevention and treatment of cancer. A plant cell thrives on carbon dioxide and gives off oxygen as its waste product. Because we are composed of animal cells, oxygen is essential for our assimilation of nutrients and the detoxification and elimination of waste products. Rational therapy must therefore include adequate oxygenation of all tissue. Other therapies prompted by Dr. Warburg's discovery must encompass all of the following in order to be effective:

1. Establish a healthy lifestyle through better nutrition, improving the personal environment and body activity.
2. The non-toxic selective destruction of cancer cells.
3. The use of antioxidants to prevent the destruction of cells by the excess production of free radicals.
4. The removal of toxic metal compounds the coat the cell's surface and interferes with normal cell respiration.
5. The support and regeneration of the immune system. The replenishment of lost or deficient nutrients (essential fatty acids, amino acids, enzymes and hormones). The elimination of all toxic accumulations.
6. Enhancement of all normal cell regeneration, particularly of the compromised tissues.
7. Psycho-immunological support for its direct effect on biochemistry.

ALL OF THESE ARE PRESENT IN THE THERAPEAUTIC PROGRAMS IN THIS BOOK.

THE FOLLOWING CHAPTERS OF THIS BOOK WILL DEAL WITH THE MANY THERAPIES OTHER THAN SURGERY, CHEMOTHERAPY AND RADIATION. THEY ARE NOT ALWAYS READILY AVAILABLE, SO I HAVE INCLUDED A LIST OF PROFESSIONAL AND ORGANIZATIONAL RESOURCES TO HELP YOU FIND THEM. I HAVE ALSO LISTED THE THERAPIES INDICATED FOR SPECIFIC TYPES OF CANCER BASED ON THE DOCUMENTATION AVAILABLE. IT FOLLOWS THE DISCUSSIONS OF EACH OF THE PRODUCTS AND METHODS SO THAT YOU WILL BE FAMILIAR WITH WHAT IS RECOMMENDED.

****

Chapter 3

Safe And Effective Therapies That Make Sense

AMYGDALIN (Leatrile, Vitamin B-17)

The most effective "medicines" and disease preventives have always been the natural substances in our environment. Invariably, it has been a deficiency in these materials which have made us vulnerable to the subsequent loss of the ability to co-exist with the environment. When a common organic substance is essential for maintaining metabolism it is classified as a vitamin. Amygdalin meets these qualifications and has been labeled vitamin B-17 by its principal investigators. **Vitamin deficiency always results in disease, and there is ample evidence to believe that cancer, at least in part, is due to a deficiency of B-17. The standard American diet (SAD) has been pitifully depleted of the foods containing B-17.** Amygdalin is not a "new drug." This designation has been applied by the FDA because it is processed in its preparation. This is done primarily because, once disease has occurred, larger amounts are needed and the purity and stability require these measures. Amygdalin was used for the treatment of tumors 3,500 years ago by the Chinese. It was prepared in its pure state in 1830 by Robiquot and Boutron. Dr. Fedor J.

Inosemzov, the prominent Russian physician, used Amygdalin successfully in 1845, in the treatment of two "fungus-like tumors."

The most cost-effective form of Amygdalin is obtained from apricot kernels and its modern formulation was discovered by Dr. Ernst T. Krebs Sr. Amygdalin is also known as Laetrile (**Lae**vomandeloni**trile**) and Vitamin B-17. It belongs to a large group of biochemical substances known as benzaldehyde cyanophoric glycosides or **nitrilosides** for short. They are comprised of molecules made up of hydrogen cyanide, a benzene ring or an acetone and a sugar. This group is non-toxic and water soluble. It is normal to the food chain of humans and animals. In fact, over 1200 plants of which 350 are edible contain these non-toxic, anti-cancer natural plant factors. The metabolic pathways of nitrilosides are fascinating and help us understand how they work against cancer. In the intestine, bacteria produce the enzyme B-glycosidase which hydrolyzes the nitrilosides and release **hydrogen cyanide, benzaldehyde** or **acetone** and **sugar**.

Hydrogen cyanide is highly lethal (cytotoxic) and is detoxified in a normal cell by the enzyme **rhodanase** to thiocyanate which is relatively non-toxic. However, a cancer cell is deficient in rhodanase production and therefore is vulnerable to the lethal effects of the cyanide.

Benzaldehyde, also a powerful cytotoxin, is rapidly **oxidized** to the non-toxic benzoic acid in the oxidative metabolism of a normal cell. In the cancer cell, it should be remembered, the metabolic pathway is fermentation, similar to that of a plant cell This was the process demonstrated by Dr Otto Warburg, for which he was awarded the Nobel Prize.

The combination of benzaldehyde and hydrogen cyanide is synergistic and exhibits a cytotoxic effect far in excess of the sum of their separate effects. Remember this basic principle of synergism everytime you read that the FDA says that another one of the carcinogens they allow is too little to cause damage. Amygdalin given orally to test animals is 1/20th as toxic as Aspirin. Compare this to the cytotoxins of the medical-pharmaceutical establishment known as chemotherapy which kills 25% of the patients on which they are used. Yet, the two compounds, benzaldehyde and hydrogen cyanide in synergy, are more powerful than any establishment chemotherapy currently in use - YET THEY ARE SAFE - because they are part of our natural food chain and our adaptation over millions of years has given us the enzymes to neutralize their effect on normal cells. Unfortunately we are being starved of the fatty acids necessary to produce enzymes (see the chapter on linseed oil).

Evidence abounds that bitter almonds, the richest source of amygdalin, has been ingested by humans for medicinal purposes for more than 2,000 years. If one adds an acetyl radical to the effective part of amygdalin, the compound formed is acetylsalicylic acid (**aspirin**). In a recent study of the prophylactic effect of aspirin on coronary heart disease involving over 600,000 volunteers, **it was coincidentally discovered that aspirin had a significant effect (50%) on reducing the incidence of cancer of the colon**. Aspirin, however, can cause serious problems, especially intestinal bleeding and even death. Its anti-cancer effects are far less than amygdalin.

Aspirin (O-hydroxybenzaldehyde) from willow and poplar bark, the benzaldehyde inclusion glucosides from figs and the nitrilosides (laetriles) from many hundreds of edible plants all are derived from non-toxic plant glucosides. They are all hydrolyzable by beta-glucosidase and metabolically produce the benzaldehyde non-sugar, **aglycone,** which is one of the biologically important ingredients. It is a mild local anesthetic and the pain relieving effect of Amygdalin is in part, likely due to the action of benzaldehyde on the nerve endings.

In spite of the antineoplastic and carcinostatic effects of this safe and effective compound, the establishment continues to employ the three very profitable, toxic, dehumanizing, often cancer-causing, ineffective and iatrogenic modalities of surgery, radiation and chemotherapy. This approach has continued for more than a half a century while the cancer death rate has tripled. The anti-cancer effect of amygdalin was demonstrated in Mexico by government sponsored research under Dr. Mario Soto De Leon and its use is legal. Dr. Soto was the first medical director of the Cydel Clinic in Tijuana. It is vitally important that it be prepared and administered correctly in sufficient dosage or it will not be effective. The trial performed at the Mayo Clinic in the early 80's involved the use of the racemic mixture rather than the levo-rotary form and thus was only at

10% of the strength required. In spite of this, toward the end of the experiment the patients began to show improvement, but it was discontinued and declared ineffectual. The "cancer cocktail" administered should follow the proven protocol containing DMSO and large doses of vitamin C. Amygdalin is continued as an oral preparation after leaving institutional care, in amounts to be determined by the physician. It must be continued for life in order to maintain its beneficial anti-cancer effects. Apricot kernels can be injested (one for each 10 to 15 pounds of body weight divided into six or more doses during the day. Example: a person weighing 120 lbs. would chew (they are bitter) 2 kernals every 2 to 3 hours during the day for a total of 12 kernals.

****

CHELATION

WHAT IS CHELATION?

Chelation therapy is probably the most significant medical discovery of this century. The benefits derived exceed that of any other single modality and extend to almost every disease known to medicine. The word chelate (pronounced key-late) is derived from the Greek "chele" meaning "claw". Crabs and lobsters are chelates. The biochemistry of the chelating agent used in this therapy is a process in which it grasps metals such as calcium, magnesium, potassium, and deadly metals like mercury and lead, and carries them out of the body without entering the body metabolism. The metabolism chelating agent, ethylene diamine tetra-acetic acid (EDTA), was first synthesized in Germany in the late 1930's for use in industry and was reported in 1952 as a treatment for lead poisoning. It remains the treatment of choice for heavy metal poisoning throughout the world. Chelation is one of the most important natural processes in nature. It makes possible the utilization of inorganic minerals by plants and animals (that includes humans). Everyone is familiar with at least two chelating agents, chlorophyll and hemoglobin (which transports oxygen), but they were probably never identified as such when you learned about them in school.

HOW DOES CHELATION WORK?

Chelation promotes health by correcting the underlying cause of arterial blockage. Oxygen free radicals are increased by the presence of metallic elements in the body. They are damaging to tissue because they act as a chronic irritant to blood vessel walls and cell membranes. EDTA removes those metallic irritants, allowing leaking and damaged cell walls to heal. This markedly improves oxygen delivery to the cell and the elimination of the waste products of metabolism from the cell. The plaques lining the walls of the arteries shrink and smooth over, thus allowing more blood to circulate. The blood vessel walls regain their elasticity and respond to changes in pressure more readily. Thousands of studies bear witness to the ability of EDTA to increase blood flow significantly. Thus Chelation is of great benefit in several ways:

1. Improves circulation, which;
2. Delivers oxygen to the cells, which;
3. Removes poisonous compounds, which;
4. Improves cell membrane transfer of nutrients and waste, which;
5. Allows for better mobilization and implementation of all defensive protective mechanisms and offensive weapons against disease and facilitates the reparative processes necessary for healing to take place.

WHAT IS CHELATION USED FOR?

The most important use of chelation has been in the treatment of atherosclerosis and arteriosclerosis. By chelating out the calcium-cholesterol plaques that occlude arterial walls, EDTA, which is administered intravenously, markedly improves circulation to every part of the body including the heart and the brain. We have all been exposed to metallic poisons most of our lives. Mercury, lead and cadmium are the most deadly. All metals can be toxic if present in excessive amounts or if they have been deposited where they don't belong. Compounds are formed that interfere with normal metabolism and promote the formation of destructive tissue changes. It immediately becomes apparent that chelation has to be beneficial in any disease in which improved circulation and the elimination of toxic substances aid in the body's ability to heal itself. Virtually every disease is in that category, without exception. Chelation has not only improved **heart disease, stroke, high blood pressure, arthritis, Parkinson's and Alzheimer's disease. Studies indicate a 50% reduction in the occurrence of cancer in individuals who have received EDTA.** Chelation has been reported to improve **asthma, emphysema, brain function, muscular coordination, Multiple Sclerosis and impotence. It also slows down the aging process** by preventing free radical damage.

HAS CHELATION BEEN FULLY TESTED AND IS IT SAFE?

More than 500,000 patients have received chelation therapy in the United States alone. It has been primarily used in coronary artery disease and peripheral occlusive vascular disease. The ability of chelation to safely improve serious heart and circulatory problems has been consistently been reported in the 90% range. The safety record for its' use has been exceptional. More than 30 million treatments have been administered without a single serious complication, except in rare instances when the standard rules of procedure were not followed and the patient is not properly evaluated. Not one single death has been directly caused by chelation therapy when administered by a properly trained physician. Compare that with the 5% - 6% death rate from bypass surgery, which does not even extend life expectancy. Today there are over one thousand scientific papers that support the many biochemical actions of EDTA and over two dozen clinical papers, including double-blind studies which support the incredible medical benefits to patients in a wide variety of conditions. There have been only two papers which have criticized the use of EDTA. These papers are based on opinion or apply to techniques which have been obsolete for decades. They come from physicians who have a vested interest in catheterization and surgery, or who have bowed to the pressures of the establishment.

IS CHELATION JUST EDTA?

In addition to EDTA, the intravenous infusions contain from five to twenty other ingredients designed to replace the good minerals which may be removed with the bad. Substantial amounts of vitamin C and other vitamins are included, as well as blood thinners and other substances, which safely enhance EDTA. Any intelligent therapy involves change in life-style and diet. Chelation is no exception! EDTA can be used in combination with almost any other therapy. It is always important for the physician to know everything the patient is taking. Chelation often eliminates the need or the reduces dosage of the medicines a patient may be taking.

CAN ANYBODY TAKE CHELATION?

The only major contraindication to chelation therapy is the presence of kidney failure. Even then, it may be possible to use it, if administered in reduced dosage, with careful monitoring.

HOW DO I KNOW IF I NEED CHELATION?

If you are from this planet you probably need it! However, chelation is most likely imperative if you are short of breath, have chest pain, leg pain while walking, transient or progressive loss of vision or memory, paralysis, poor circulation, gangrene, diabetes or any disease for that matter. For all of these symptoms or conditions, and even if you have had by-pass surgery and would like to avoid one, two, or three more death-defying leaps into the operating room, then SEE A PHYSICIAN THAT DOES CHELATION IMMEDIATELY! IT IS LEGAL IN MANY STATES IN THE U.S. for use in cardiovascular disease and even cancer. Even though chelation therapy is recognized world-wide for mercury and lead poisoning, its use in cancer and other degenerative diseases places the administering physician under great risk of harassment and loss of license. Why? It is a serious threat to the twelve billion dollar-a-year - 95% over-utilized, non-life extending and deadly cardiovascular surgical industry.

IS CHELATION USEFUL IN TREATING CANCER?

Many clinics in Europe, Mexico and South America, use chelation in the treatment of cancer. Simple logic dictates that any therapy which improves the general circulation is likely to be useful in the treatment of any disease, particularly in cancer. This is not to imply that it has a direct effect on cancer cells. Walter Blumer, M.D. and Elmer M. Cranton, M.D., in the Journal of Advancement In Medicine, Volume 2, 1989 presented an 18-year follow-up study on 59 patients that had been treated with calcium-EDTA (chelation). The study evaluated the incidence of mortality from cancer. They reported that only one of the 59 patients died of cancer during this period. This represented only 1.7%. A control group of 172 individuals from the same area was evaluated and the incidence of cancer was 17.6%. (30 out of 172 persons died of cancer). **This is a 90% reduction in cancer mortality for the chelation treated group.** A careful statistical analysis failed to reveal any other factors which were different between the two groups - CHELATION WAS THE ONLY DIFFERENCE! I think it is safe to say that anything that prevents, is likely to help in treatment.

WHAT IS THE COST?

Chelation usually costs $2,000 to $6,000 for 20 to 40 treatments. Every cell and every artery in the body is safely benefited, while in by-pass surgery less than one inch of an artery is removed at mortal risk. By-pass surgery is usually more than $40,000 dollars, does nothing for the rest of your body and does not extend your life. I think we are all worth the price of a used car!

In the past fifty years literally tens of thousands of pages have been written in the thousands of journals published each year in the United States alone, exposing many factors in our diet which are deadly. Much of this important information has been published in books and government documents. The news media has headlined this information from time to time. But, while we continue to bring poisons to our lips at every meal each day, the National Cancer Institute, the American Cancer Society, the F.D.A. and the Congress of the United States pay "lip service" and do nothing to protect us. We have armies and police to protect our lives and property. There are laws which protect us from reckless drivers, pollution, murder and mayhem. The FDA is preventing health food companies from placing information on labels of vitamins, minerals and supplements indicating what research has disclosed with reference to probable benefits. When it comes to processed food, however, they do not require that information about the harmful effects of the processing be placed on the label. This is typical FDA "fairness".

****

CHELATION PROTOCOLS

The protocol outlined is the basic protocol recommended by The American College of Advancement in Medicine (see referrence section).

1. **Sterile H2O, Ringer's lactate, saline, or 5% glucose solution** - 1,000 cc
2. **EDTA** (ethylene diamine tetra-acetic acid) - 3gm (range of 50mg/kg of body wt. - max. 5gm)
3. **Magnesium** - 3ml of 50% MgSO4
4. **Procaine or Lidocaine (2%)** - 5 to 10cc (max. 20cc) - procaine is preferable but more allergenic)
5. **Heparin** - 1,000 to 5,000 units (not to be used if patient is already anticoagulated)
6. **Ascorbate** - 4gm to 20gm of Vitamin C
7. **Potassium** - 10mEq to 20mEq of KCl (5-10cc)
8. **Hydrochloric Acid** - 20 to 40mg HCl (2-5cc)
9. **Pyridoxine** - 100mg to 300mg (1-3cc)
10. **Dexpanthenol** - 250mg to 750 mg (1-3cc) Supplementary I.V (given as a "piggy-back" drip during the last 20cc of the standard infusion), along with additional:

   a. Ascorbate, 5cc
   b. Dexpanthenol, 1-3ccc.
   c. Pyrodoxine, 1cc
   d. Vitamin B12, 1cc
   e. Niacinamide, 1cc
   f. B-complex 2-5cc
   g. Trace Minerals, 1cc

NOTE:

VARIATIONS OF THE INGREDIENTS OTHER THAN EDTA ARE USED DEPENDING UPON THE CONDITION BEING TREATED AND THE COEXISTING DISEASES OF THE PATIENT. THIS IS WHY SPECIAL TRAINING IS REQUIRED AND A PHYSICIAN WHO IS A MEMBER OF THE AMERICAN COLLEGE FOR ADVANCES IN MEDICINE (OPEN TO PHYSICIANS OF ALL COUNTRIES) IS RECOMMENDED.

****

Chapter 4

The Breath Of Life

OZONE (O3) "Breath of God" (ancient Hebrew)
CANCER CELLS CANNOT SURVIVE IN AN OXYGEN
RICH ENVIRONMENT!
"The prime cause of cancer is the replacement of normal
oxygen respiration of body cells by an anaerobic (lacking in
oxygen) cell respiration."
Dr. Otto Warburg, twice a Nobel Laureate

NOTE: THE USE OF OZONE THERAPY IN THE TREAT-
MENT OF CANCER OR ANY OTHER DISEASE IS
UNPROVEN AND NOT RECOGNIZED BY THE FDA OR
THE MEDICAL PROFESSION IN THE UNITED STATES.
THIS CHAPTER PRESENTS INFORMATION ABOUT ITS
HISTORY AND HOW IT IS BEING USED BY THOUSANDS
OF PRACTITIONERS THROUGHOUT THE WORLD. ONLY
34 CASES OF SIDE EFFECTS OUT OF 5,500,000 PATIENTS
HAVE BEEN REPORTED.

ABOUT OZONE
The discovery and naming of ozone is attributed to Christian
Friedrich Schonbein in 1840. It's value in medicine was debated
for many decades and references to its use were sporadic. Dr.
Albert Wolf, a German physician wrote in 1915. "As regards
the medical usability of ozone, the viewpoint of experimental
science may be considered as being in direct opposition to the

practical experiences gained by industry." He used ozone successfully in the treatment of decubitus ulcers. During the First World War (1915) ozone gas was used to help the healing of serious wounds. Ozone has been used to purify the drinking water of major cities since 1901. The first was Vienna and the most recent was Los Angeles. It does not give water the disagreeable taste that chlorine does. Although many authorities refer to it as poisonous and a hazard to life, like anything else on this planet, if used properly it is beneficial - in fact life would become extinct without ozone in our atmosphere. The breathing of inappropriate concentrations is indeed harmful to the lungs, but in proper concentrations it purifies the air we breath. Home and industrial ozonators are used throughout the world (including the United States, to purify the air), and yet, comments are being made publicly by authoritative figures that ozone is poisonous and a hazard to life. This is indeed true if, as in the case of any substance on this earth, it is used in unsafe amounts. Statements of this nature are unjustified and fraudulent when they are intended to misinform or alarm the public in a way that would indicate that ozone is unsafe under any circumstances.

Ozone is created by the action of ultraviolet light or a strong electrical field on oxygen atoms. The result is the forcing together of 3 atoms into unstable groups (O_3) that rather quickly break down into the usual oxygen molecule (O_2). Ozone is lethal to almost all viruses, bacteria, fungus and cancer cells. The scientific literature is replete with articles proving these facts.

Ozone is formed in our atmosphere naturally by the effect of lightning on oxygen. It is that wonderful sweet smell that you can detect after a summer storm. It is nature's method of cleansing our atmosphere of contamination. The poisonous ozone levels reported effecting our cities differs dramatically in that it represents the combining of the extensive overwhelming pollution with ozone insufficient to do the job. If you wonder why cancer rates have tripled in the last 20 years, consider this startling fact:

Oxygen represented 36% of the air we breathed 200 years ago. Today it is only 19%! (From the work of La Voisier - the discoverer of oxygen and current figures)

In 1931, Dr. Otto Warburg was awarded the Nobel Prize in biochemistry. Dr. Warburg demonstrated that the metabolism of a cancer cell was like that of a plant cell, which thrives on carbon dioxide and gives off oxygen as its waste product. It actually represents the process of fermentation. We are composed of animal cells and oxygen is essential for our assimilation of nutrients and the detoxification and elimination of waste products. When ozone is introduced into the bloodstream, it is converted into oxygen, hydroxyperoxides and other beneficial free radical scavengers which actually seek out and destroy diseased cells.

Nearly 50 years later, the prestigious journal SCIENCE, VOL. 209, 22 AUGUST 1980, published a paper entitled: OZONE SELECTIVELY INHIBITS GROWTH OF HUMAN CANCER CELLS. This paper dealt with the exposure of human lung, breast and uterine cancer, tissue to ozone at concentrations of 0.3 to 0.8 parts per million, well within the non-toxic limits (OSHA standards). More than 1,000 parts per million can be tolerated safely during the average ten minute period that medically administered ozone takes and concentrations far less than that are used. In the experiments, normal human cells were not effected at these levels. The modern development of ozone application in medicine gained impetus in the 1950's in Europe, and its use gradually spread throughout Europe to Australia, Israel and Brazil.

INTRA-VENOUS OZONE GAS is extremely safe and effective against all infections. The earliest evidence that I could locate, of ozone's recommendation as therapy in the United States, appeared in an 1885 issue of the Journal of the Dade County Medical Association. In spite of this and many other references prior to 1920, the FDA has illegally raided and confiscated ozone generators from the offices of advanced (alternative) physicians.

Ozone is classified as a toxic gas if inhaled in large quantities. However, it is not toxic when injected slowly into the body by intra-arterial injections, I.V., intramuscularly, subcutaneously or by vaginal or rectal insufflation. Ozone has no side effects when administered, using these methods, in the proper quantities and concentrations. It does not effect healthy cells of any type adversely under those conditions.

It is obvious why it is lethal to cancer cells. The cancer (plant) cell is being given its toxic waste product, while our normal cells are being given their essential for life. Individuals receiving ozone for the first time are usually apprehensive. It is scary to have "air" injected into their veins. They have images of dying from an air embolus. Almost everyone seems to recollect a murder mystery in which the villain killed his victim that way in the hopes of committing the perfect crime. It will never happen in real life because:

1. Nitrogen would have to be present in order to cause a toxic reaction and therapeutically only pure medical grade oxygen is used.

2. It would take at least 50 cc of gas given within 2 to 3 seconds. That can't even be accomplished with a very large bore 18 gauge needle. The procedure is done with a tiny 25 gauge needle. Death could only occur intentionally, never accidentally.

Specific therapeutic applications of ozone include the treatment of circulatory problems, decubitus ulcers, **some forms of cancer** (still under investigation as to how many), AIDS, viral diseases, wounds, scars, burns, gangrene and liver disease including hepatitis. Ozone is the only substance known which is a virucidal, bactericidal, fungicidal, protozoacidal and cancericidal. Over 1000 medical papers exist in the world medical literature attesting to its efficacy in the treatment of disease in many tens of thousands of patients. Typically it has been ignored in America because it can't be patented. Therefore it is not profitable for the pharmaceutical industry to spend the millions of dollars necessary to prove its effectiveness by FDA standards. It would reap scorn and outrage of incredible proportions if the truth were known. The pharmaceutical industry and the FDA confuse and distort the role of ozone in our ecosystem and suppress its use therapeutically (even though, under law, it should be "grandfathered in").

In addition to the many articles on the use of ozone in medicine, there are medical texts such as "THE USE OF OZONE IN MEDICINE" by Prof. Siegfried Rilling, M.D. and Renate Viebahn, Ph. D., and medical organizations in the major industrial nations of the world dedicated to the education and instruction of its use.

A WORLD OF OZONE CONFERENCE has been held frequently since the early 1970's, the most recent was held in San Francisco (1993). and was attended by hundreds of doctors from many countries. Russia sent seven scientists to present papers on their discoveries of its application. In no other science does acceptance take as long as it does in medicine. The use of deep freezing techniques took over 80 years and television over 30 years, but in medicine, where human life is at stake, it can take 150 years and maybe never if there is no profit to be made. Fortunately for mankind, there are still countries where investigation into non-drug, non-patentable, non-toxic and inexpensive therapies are still being carried out.

SUBSTANTIAL EVIDENCE

The PROCEEDINGS OF THE WORLD OZONE CONFERENCES have documented and published the techniques and dosages of ozone for its beneficial use in the following conditions:

Cancer (Carcinoma)	SpasticColon	Acne
Osteomyelitis	Acne	Proctitis
Bladder Fistula	Wounds, Ulcers	Varicosities
Radiation burns	Phlebitises	Parkinson's
Ulcerative Colitis	Mucous Colitis	Chronic Cystitis
Colitis	Parkinsons	Coli Infections
Chronic Hepatitis	Hemorrhoids	Anal Eczema
Arterial Thrombosis	Arthritis	

Intrarectal insufflation is excellent for diarrhea and candidiasis (in women **intravaginal insufflation** is also effective), and it is applied in this manner when intravenous administration is impractical or unavailable.

As long as the lobbyists and influence peddlers for the pharmaceutical industry and the AMA are able to convince our representatives that anything outside of the mainstream of medicine is either useless, fraudulent or dangerous, many safe, non-toxic and effective therapies will be denied to the public. Our representatives must be made aware that although the safety is not usually the problem, proof of efficacy by the double-blind standard is economically prohibitive. In those instances where such proof has been offered, fraudulent tactics by the opposition have resulted in blocking the use of some incredible therapies (see the chapters on Amygdalin and chelation).

If you want to know what benefits ozone bestows in disease, ask the doctors and patients who have used it - but, of course, that's anecdotal!!!

THE IMPORTANCE OF OXYGEN

Virtually every patient's room in a modern hospital is equipped for the administration of oxygen. Certainly, an emergency room cannot be without one because it is required by law. Deep breathing exercises are prescribed for patients with lung problems and for individuals recovering from surgery. The narrow use of these techniques are indeed unfortunate. they should be routine for all patients. The local gymnasiums and health spas routinely employ the proper use of deep breathing exercises. The average person takes their respiration for granted. The are large religious cults who incorporate consciousness of breathing as an important ritual of their beliefs. Indians refer to "Prana" as a wonderful substance that God has provided for a healthy life. Certainly, Prana is oxygen, or possibly even ozone. Both aptly fit their description. Obviously, deep breathing exercises carry greater importance today, because of the lowered concentration in our atmosphere, than ever before. The effect of gradual oxygen deprivation on metabolism is devastating and leads to an inadequate processing of the toxic wastes that our bodies are constantly producing. One of the consequences of lowered oxygen concentration is the elevation of uric acid in the body. This one compound alone, is implicated in a wide variety of metabolic problems. The most common disease associated with a uric acid disorder is gout and it is primarily due to an inability to process meat protein. However, the far reaching effects on almost every system of the body gives us an indication of the widespread effect that a low-grade increase can have. The formation of a stone in the kidneys and gallbladder, the blocking of circulation and the destruction of joints by the formation of crystals are just a few of the problems that arise. There are literally hundreds of known biochemical reactions in the body that utilize oxygen. There are probably many thousands more waiting to be discovered. Acute deprivation of oxygen leads to a rapid death. We are getting there more quickly than we should. The importance of oxidative processes is discussed more fully elsewhere, but the relationship with the development and progress of cancer is no longer in doubt. The use of ozone appears to go beyond the benefit of oxygen in the treatment of disease. The production of electromagnetic energy at the molecular level, as the ozone molecule disassociates into oxygen, undoubtedly plays a role in its usefulness in therapy. Permit me to list just a few of the proven effects of ozone.

OZONE ACTIONS

1. OZONE ACTIVATES THE ENZYMES INVOLVED IN PEROXIDE OR OXYGEN "FREE RADICAL" DESTRUCTION i.e. GLUTATHIONE, CATALASE, S.O.D.
2. ACCELERATES GLYCOLYSIS (BREAKDOWN OF GLYCOGEN) IN RBCs, THUS IT:
   a. INCREASES THE RELEASE OF O_2 FROM THE HEMOGLOBIN IN THE BLOOD TO THE TISSUES.
   b. ENHANCES FORMATION OF ACETYL CO-ENZYME- A, WHICH IS VITAL IN METABOLIC DETOXIFICATION.
   c. INFLUENCES THE MITOCHONDRIAL TRANSPORT SYSTEM WHICH ENHANCES THE METABOLISM OF ALL CELLS AND SAFEGUARDS AGAINST MUTAGENIC CHANGES.
   d. INCREASES RED BLOOD CELL PLIABILITY, BLOOD FLUIDITY AND ARTERIAL pO_2 (OXYGEN CONTENT) AND A DECREASE IN ROULEAUX FORMATION (CLUMPING) WHICH INTERFERES WITH THE NORMAL FUNCTIONING OF RED BLOOD CELL METABOLISM.
3. INCREASES LEUKOCYTOSIS (PRODUCTION OF WHITE BLOOD CELLS) AND PHAGOCYTOSIS (THE MANNER IN WHICH CERTAIN WHITE BLOOD

CELLS DESTROY FOREIGN MATTER). BOTH PROCESSES ARE PART OF THE IMMUNE DEFENSE SYSTEM.

4. STIMULATES THE RETICULO - ENDOTHELIAL SYSTEM, THE REBUILDING OF TISSUE.
5. STRONG GERMICIDE - INACTIVATES ENTEROVIRUSES, COLIFORM BACTERIA, SAPHY-LOCOCCUS AUREUS AND AEROMONA HYDROPHI-LIA.
6. DISRUPTS THE CELL ENVELOPE OF MANY PATHOGENIC ORGANISMS WHICH ARE COM-POSED OF PHOSPHOLIPIDS, PEPTIDOGLYCANS AND POLYSACCHARIDES.
7. OPENS THE CIRCULAR PLASMID DNA WHICH LESSENS BACTERIAL PROLIFERATION.
8. FUNGICIDAL, INHIBITS CANDIDA CELL GROWTH.
9. LOW DOSES STIMULATE THE IMMUNE SYSTEM
10. HIGH DOSES INHIBIT THE IMMUNE SYSTEM
11. LIMIT DOSE TO 3,000 ug.

References: The information for this chapter is culled from the hundreds of papers presented at the World Conferences on Ozone. The scarcity of information available in the major medical journals is testimony to the power of the Pharmaceutical industry. With good reason, they have established a wall of silence and welcome the dissemination of falsehoods about the effects of ozone. They have an entire market of antibiotics at stake. There is no evidence that anyone has ever died from ozone therapy, and my conversations with practitioners in several countries, including the United States, confirms the remarkable results that I observed first-hand in my own practice.

CRYOGENIC CELL THERAPY

THE INCREDIBLE FACTS OF LIFE AND CELL THERAPY:

CELL THERAPY IS SAFE.
CELL THERAPY IS EFFECTIVE.
CELL THERAPY HAS BEEN THOROUGHLY TESTED

CELL THERAPY IS IN USE THROUGHOUT THE WORLD.
CELL THERAPY HAS BEEN PROVEN USEFUL IN ALMOST EVERY DISEASE CATEGORY INCLUDING:

CANCER, CARDIOVASCULAR DISEASE, GENETIC DISEASES, DEGENERATIVE DISEASES, NEUROLOGICAL DISORDERS, SKIN DISEASES, IMMUNOLOGICAL PROBLEMS, HORMONAL AND GLANDULAR DISEASES AND IN REJUVENATION, REGENERATION & REVITALIZATION.

CELL THERAPY IS BEING USED BY MORE THAN **FIFTY THOUSAND PHYSICIANS** THROUGHOUT THE WORLD

CELL THERAPY HAS BEEN ADMINISTERED TO WELL OVER **TWO MILLION INDIVIDUALS** INCLUDING POPE PIUS XII, PRESIDENT AND MAMIE EISENHOWER, WINSTON CHURCHILL, THE DUKE AND DUCHESS OF WINDSOR, CHARLES CHAPLIN AND COUNTLESS OTHER CELEBRITIES.

CELL THERAPY CAN BE TRACED AS FAR BACK AS 1550 B.C. (EBER PAPYRUS). CELL THERAPY BY MODERN INJECTION TECHNIQUES WAS FIRST REPORTED IN 1912 BY KUTTNER.

YET...

CELL THERAPY IS CONSIDERED "UNPROVEN" AND THEREFORE ILLEGAL IN THE UNITED STATES OF AMERICA

IN PERSPECTIVE

The history of cell therapy is fascinating and extremely educational. There are thousands of books. newspaper and magazine articles, research papers and medical documents establishing cell therapy's long and extensive use and applications. Consider for example, that even cannibalism, when it was thoroughly investigated, revealed beliefs attributing therapeutic powers to the various specific parts of the body when ingested.

Modern cell therapy owes its current popularity to the brilliant work of Dr. Paul Niehans, a Swiss surgeon who is considered the "Father of Cellular therapy". Dr. Niehans' research revealed that embryonic (fetal) tissue of other mammals did not elicit a rejection reaction in humans because the tissue was so primitive that it had not yet developed **antigenicity** (before the maternal immune response was in place). That simply meant that the tissue at an early fetal stage had not differentiated to the point where it could be distinguished from human tissue by the body's immune defenses. It therefore could be assimilated by human tissue as its own without being rejected and destroyed.

We have all read of experiments that have been carried out using a Pig's liver as a transplant for a human. It is only through the use of dangerous immune suppressives that even temporary success can be obtained. We are equally aware that transplanting organs from one human to another is only sometimes successfully accomplished with extreme difficulty and too often with great peril to the recipient. A logical individual would at least try safe fetal tissue injections early in the disease, but when has the FDA (Food and Drug Administration or sometimes affectionately referred to as the "Federal Damnation Administration") and the Medical establishment ever acted logically?

The irrefutable evidence that cellular injections existed prior to the FDA regulations proscribing the use of new untested therapies, places it in the category referred to as being "grandfathered in". There are many articles in the establishment American medical literature supporting the use of cellular therapy, especially in some deadly diseases of children. However, the FDA, in the interest of protecting the enormously profitable "drug culture" of the pharmaceutical industry and allopathic (establishment) medicine, has violated the directives of the U.S. Congress. Sadly, our representatives are snowed by the powerful lobbyists of the AMA and the Pharmaceutical Industry "Syndicate" (PIS). Most representatives are not knowledgeable in medical science and innocently believe what they hear as the Gospel.

Cellular therapy cannot be patented and therefore poses a serious economic threat to the pharmaceutical industry. It becomes obvious why the AMA, the FDA and the PIS constantly divert the public's attention to the discovery of synthetic drugs, hormones and enzymes rather than the widespread availability of the inexpensive and safer naturally occurring substances. All this, while millions suffer and die. There are some circumstances, as in diabetes, where only human embryonic cells are effective and when injected into the muscle of juvenile diabetics, negate the need for daily multiple injections for periods of a year or more. The current disputes over the use of human embryonic tissue, if settled intelligently, promises to alleviate the terrible suffering endured by millions in a variety of diseases. Genetic engineering also is very promising, but what about the millions who need help now?

Since the death of Niehans in 1971, many research scientists have advanced and continued his work. Wolfram W. Kunhau, M.D., has expanded the field of hormone therapy and by discovering the relationship of centers of the brain that play a vital role in hormone production.

HOW CELL THERAPY WORKS

When very young fetal cells are injected into muscle tissue, they migrate by genetic coding (biochemical, physiological and bio-electrical properties) which enable these cells to recognize and integrate with their corresponding tissue in the body. Experiments, laboratory tests, practical observation and experience has provided irrefutable evidence that these cells revitalize the old cells and restore organ function for very long periods of time. The implications of what can be and has been achieved are enormous. With regard to disease, just the role of Thymus tissue alone evokes the possibility of at least a thousand possible applications. This important organ of immune defense begins to falter and atrophy rather early in life, leaving us progressively at the mercy of aging and the increased occurrence of all disease. This important organ tissue when injected synergistically with Mesenchyme, Hypothalamus and others, provide an important boost in the body's fight against cancer and most diseases.

INDICATIONS
(A complete list of the individual diseases would fill pages)

- IMMUNE DEFICIENCY DISEASES
- MOST CANCERS
- GENERAL LOSS OF VITALITY
- GLANDULAR IMPAIRMENT
- REDUCED INTELLECTUAL FUNCTION
- IMPOTENCE & STERILITY
- CENTRAL NERVOUS SYSTEM DYSFUNCTION & DEGENERATION (ALZHHEIMER'S, PARKINSON'S, etc.)
- ALL ARTHRITIS
- DIABETES MELLITIS
- CHRONIC SKIN DISEASES (ECZEMA, PSORIASIS)
- FEMALE HORMONE DEFICIENCY (MENOPAUSE, STERILITY)
- THYROID PROBLEMS
- PMS
- SKIN (DECUBITUS) ULCERS
- OSTEOPOROSIS
- CIRCULATORY INSUFFICIENCY (EYES, EXTREM-
- ITIES, HIGH OR LOW BLOOD PRESSURE etc.)
- DOWN'S SYNDROME (MONGOLOIDISM)
- ALL DEGENERATIVE DISEASES
- LIVER & GALL BLADDER DISEASES (CIRRHOSIS)
- DEPRESSED STATES (NEURO-VEGETATIVE DISORDERS)
- GROWTH DISTURBANCES IN THE YOUNG
- PANCREATIC DISEASES
- INTESTINAL DISEASES
- SPINE, JOINT & BONE DISEASES
- COLON DISEASES
- MOST BACK PROBLEMS
- CHRONIC INFECTIONS OF THE RESPIRATORY SYSTEM
- DIGESTIVE PROBLEMS

- CHILDREN'S HEREDITARY OR ACQUIRED BRAIN DISEASE
- CHRONIC LUNG DISEASE

CONTRAINDICATIONS TO CELL THERAPY

- ACUTE INFECTIONS
- CONTINUING ANTICOAGULANT THERAPY
- ACUTE INFLAMMATION
- RECURRENT THROMBOSIS OR EMBOLISM
- ACUTE HEART PROBLEMS
- CHRONIC KIDNEY DISEASE/DYSFUNCTION (ELEVATED CREATININE)
- CEREBRAL HEMORRHAGE
- SEVERE HYPERTENSION
- GOUT - HIGH URIC ACID
- HEPATITIS
- HEMOPHILIA
- ALLERGY TO VACCINES, SERA OR DRUGS

CELL PREPARATION AND ADMINISTRATION

Sixty years of modern use, research and experimentation has resulted in the application of the miraculous technique of Cryogenics to cell therapy. This historical discovery has enabled medical science to preserve tissue for extremely long periods, in a state of suspended animation. Preservation of live sperm, tissue and bone banks and ultra-safe cell therapy are but a few of the benefits. The technique involves the flash-freezing of live cells at minus one hundred and sixty degrees centigrade. Though there are still a few advocates of live cells being transferred directly from the calf embryo to the patient within thirty minutes, there is no evidence that there is any advantage and the risk of infection and serious reactions are greater.

THERAPEUTIC ADMINISTRATION
OF THE CELLS

Physician Procedures:
(All of the Following information is to be related to the patient

47

at least one week prior to the procedure)

    A. History and physical examination.

    B. Evaluation of clinical laboratory tests (Complete blood count, sed rate, SMAC-24 and urinalysis.

    C. Selection of cells to be used in disease.*

    D. Selection of cells for rejuvenation.**

    E. Inject cells deeply using procaine and a 21 gauge 1.5" needle, into the upper outer quadrant of the gluteus maximus muscle.

    F. Patient is instructed to have **complete bed rest for two days** and mostly rest on the third day.

Patient Instructions:

    G. Take 10 grams of Vitamin C (10,000mg) daily, individed doses for at least Five (5) days prior to therapy and Ten (10) days following therapy. This improves the health of the capillaries and cell utilization.

    H. Total bed rest except for bathroom privileges. Meals are best served in bed.

    I. Avoid exercise for ten (10) days following therapy.

    J. Avoid smoking, alcohol, antibiotics, X-rays, hot baths and sunshine for at least ten days after therapy.

    K. Reactions occur in less than one out of twenty. They are usually mild and may include: Fever, local swelling, flushing, itching and soreness.

Within approximately one week an increase in vitality may be noticed, followed by a gradual improvement in vigor, sex drive, emotional outlook, appearance, alertness and appetite.

* BASIC CELLS to be included: HYPOTHALAMUS, THYMUS, MESENCHYME, PLACENTA (male or female as appropriate) plus CELLS APPROPRIATE TO THE PROBLEM.

** USE BASIC CELLS plus CELLS INDICATED BY THE EVALUATION OF THOSE SYSTEMS MOST IN NEED. AS MANY AS EIGHT TO TEN INJECTIONS (some injections may contain more than one type of cell, often adjacent or connecting tissues, so as not to confuse the macrophages.)

Chapter 5

"Let Your Food Be Your Medicine"

Linseed - The Incredible Oil

"Linseed oil can prevent and even treat cancer successfully." The response of the average physician to this statement is always a smirk of disbelief, followed by a mocking smile. Most individuals, if they have heard of linseed oil, automatically think of paints in which it is used extensively. Today, because of the extensive, inaccurate propaganda about oils, fats, fatty acids and cholesterol, the sound of these words impart an ominous feeling. Unfortunately the public is still not aware that cholesterol is **not** the culprit. The processed and heated oils with which our diets abound, cause the cholesterol to thicken and precipitate in the blood and create circulatory problems. The choice of oils would be important if they were cold pressed, fresh and not processed. Currently our supermarkets offer only poisonous processed oils which deprive us of the essential fatty acids. However, oils are not readily available in their natural state except in some health food stores. The best sources are in Germany, and there are importers bringing it in. Production has recently begun in the United States and with popular support it will hopefully revolutionize the food industry.

I am convinced it is a useful cancer preventative and treatment.

I first became aware of the biochemical importance of linolenic and gamma-linoleic acid in metabolism less than ten years ago. The advanced medical organizations interested in more natural ways of preventing and treating disease were the first to take note of them. Organized medicine has yet to wake up to their extreme importance. Their role in oxidation and the formation of free radicals is still an enigma to most physicians. I seriously doubt that more than a handful prescribe their use or even know about them. When you develop the "drug habit" of the average physician it's hard to get away from prescribing prescription drugs. Most doctors would rather endanger their patients with "side effects" than recommend something safe, effective and natural that could be purchased without their Latin scriblings. After all, too many patients would still feel cheated if a doctor gave them good advice and then told them to go to a health food store. The public is getting wiser and someday the doctors will kick the "drug habit".

The number of medical papers dealing with the essential fatty acids probably number well over several thousand. Many are esoteric and difficult to understand. However, there are literally hundreds that deal directly with their application in everyday life, especially in the prevention and treatment of cancer. In order to give you an idea of what is available to physicians, I will mention a few of them. But first, a brief explanation. Fats make up a large part of our diet and a lot of mis-information has been disseminated about them. Natural fats are rarely a problem, in fact they are necessary in our diet. Fats are made up of groups of fatty acids, some of which are saturated and others unsaturated. According to their chemical structure, they are further divided into two groups: the omega-3 and the omega-6 fatty acids. Although several of the fatty acids are extremely important in maintaining health, our attention will be focused on the omega-3 linolenic acid and the omega-6 linoleic acids. More will be said later, but lets look at just a few of the articles that have been published.

H. W. Renner (1990) wrote about the effect of fatty acids in protecting us from cancer producing substances (mutagenics) especially the harmful cancer producing effect of the "anti-cancer" **thio-tepa**. You read it right!

A. Norman wrote on the use of a linoleic compound, sodium linoleate and its anti-tumor activity.

M.W. Pariza and Ha YL wrote extensively about linoleic acid and its **anti-carcinogenic action.**

G.A. Pritchard wrote of the benefits of the fatty acids in breast cancer (1989), as did Fritsche and Johnston in 1990.

As far back as 1980, the brilliant D.F. Horrobin, discussed the reversibility of **cancer** with fatty acids and other natural substances.

F. Fujiwara related the use of linolenic acid in neuroblastomas (1987). In 1990, Brushima confirmed his work.

N. Dipperaar wrote of the use of linolenic acid in relation to hepatoma and;

W.P. Leary wrote of its use in esophageal cancer.

L. Kaiser, in Nutrition and Cancer, in 1989, pointed out the lower incidence of breast cancer in populations that consumed larger amounts of fish.

E. E. Deschner showed us that essential fatty acids played a protective role against colon tumors. Cancer, 1990.

Robinson in Rheumatoid Disease Clinics of North America, 1991 discussed the positive effects of essential fatty acids in auto immune diseases.

In 1991, Gardiner and Duncan published a paper on the benefits of linolenic acid in **malignant melanoma,** one of the most deadly cancers - and so on.

Other articles deal with how the essential fatty acids are very effective in treating such diverse problems as: overweight and underweight, premenstrual tension, Diabetes, vascular disease, etc. It makes you wonder why the FDA permits the continuation of 80% of the therapies used in medicine which have never been subject to scientific testing standards, they are "grandfathered in" under their regulations. With the same breath however, they then refuse health food and vitamin companies from claiming therapeutic benefits from the use of many supplements, herbs, homeopathics, vitamins and minerals, even though some have been used in these diseases for thousands of years. It appears that they protect with one hand and taketh away with the other. Why don't they at least allow something like:

"Though this product has never been subject to modern standards of efficacy, it has been used for many years in the

treatment of ... "

OR

"This product has been thought to be useful in ... However, these claims have not been proven scientifically."

THEN, YOU COULD MAKE YOUR OWN DECISION! DEMAND IT, THEY ARE PAID BY YOU TO SERVE <u>YOU!</u>

The name of Dr. Johanna Budwig came up in a conversation about fatty acids with one of my colleagues in 1991. His praise of her program was so enthusiastic, I knew that I had to one day meet this remarkable woman. The opportunity to visit her presented itself finally at the end of August 1993. While completing the writing of this book and two others in magical Lanzarote, one of the beautiful Canary Islands of Spain off the coast of Morocco. I traveled to Germany for one week. It is an experience so very important, that I wish to share it with you.

****

A VISIT WITH DR. JOHANNA BUDWIG

The scientific research and writings of Dr. Johanna Budwig proved to be the most exciting discovery during my odyssey in search of answers to the cancer menace. Her work provided the scientific explanation that joined together all of the therapies that appeared to have a distinct beneficial effect in the treatment and prevention of cancer. Over forty years ago Dr. Budwig presented clear and convincing evidence, which has been confirmed by hundreds of other related scientific research papers since, that the essential fatty acids were at the core of the answer to the cancer problem. I felt compelled to travel to Germany and visit her personally so that I would have the very latest information to include in this book. I did so in early August of 1993, just prior to completing the final version of my manuscript. This brilliant pharmacist-chemist-physicist helped me understand why certain therapies, which in my own clinical experience as a physician, as well as that of the many other physicians I have talked with, truly seemed to be beneficial. I would like to share with you the knowledge gained from our talks as well as conversations that I fortuitously had with another physician with impeccable credentials and reputation.

Dr. Johanna Budwig is an extremely intelligent woman with strong convictions and a quick mind. She appears and acts at least fifteen years younger than her stated age of eighty-five. She held many positions of authority, especially as an advisor to government and industry. Her research soon led her to be at odds with the powerful food (fats and oils) industry and their allies in government. Several court cases were forced upon her by these influential interests, but she prevailed in all of them.

In the over thirty-three years that she has instructed patients in her program, she has taught many other physicians from most major countries of the world her method of treating cancer and other chronic diseases. She claims great success for her treatment and believes that any failures that have occurred were due to non-compliance with her program. She also expressed regret that many practitioners have altered the program in order to make it easier for the patient, thus diminishing chances for a successful outcome. Because I was a physician, she insisted on devoting most of our discussion to the research and principles behind the treatment that has gained her the world-wide reputation as the "linseed oil lady". It is said with affection and gratitude by cancer survivors around the world, but with disdain by her detractors in establishment medicine. On the surface, one can understand the scepticism of many physicians that a single food could have such a profound effect on a disease as diverse, ubiquitous and deadly as cancer. It is for this reason that I was anxious to explore the scientific explanations behind its use. I will present the complex bio-chemistry and physics in a manner that will hopefully make it as clear and compelling as it should be. Throughout this book, the many scientific papers published supporting the practical application of Dr. Budwig's therapy are be cited. In addition, I discuss the vital effects of the essential fatty acids on many other conditions which help you understand their critical importance. You will come to your own conclusions as to why this simple effective prevention and therapy has not only been ignored - it has been suppressed!

THE LIGHT OF TRUTH

The discoveries of Einstein, Planck, De Broglie and Kenneth Ford are linked by the work of Dr. Budwig to the Nobel Prize discoveries of Dr. Otto Warburg in cancer. Warburg believed that when we learned how to stop the development of the fermentation metabolism of cancer cells the cancer problem would be solved. Warburg understood that fats had to play a role in the process, but he was unable to discover the way in which sufficient electromagnetic force was provided for the reaction. He experimented with butyric acid, a **saturated** fatty acid which lacks the "pi-electrons" (electrons possessing particular qualities attributed to their position and behavior) which are indispensable for the transfer of oxygen. Butyric acid therefore failed to stimulate the absorption of oxygen, the necessary substance needed to destroy the cancer process.

Warburg wrote that he could not explain why he was unable to achieve the "desired and expected effect of respiration stimulation". He was referring to the fact that the chemical reactions involved in oxidation, that he expected to take place in cell metabolism, simply were not happening. It is precisely this question that Dr. Budwig has answered in her work. It took quantum physics to provide the mechanism by which the energy needed in biochemical process of oxidation would implicate the unsaturated fatty acids as the most likely provider of oxygen transport in and out of the cell. As you might recall, from high school chemistry, electrons are tiny particles that have an electrical charge and the revolve around the nucleus of an atom just like the planets revolve around the sun. It is the number of electrons in orbit, their speed and distance from the nucleus that determines what the properties of that atom will be. The chemical compounds of our bodies contain atoms of almost every substance in the universe. The most common of which are very familiar to you i.e. oxygen, hydrogen, carbon, potassium, sodium, chloride and magnesium. It is the unique combinations of these atoms, plus many more, that make up everything in our bodies including each enzyme, hormone amd every type of tissue of which we are composed. The way in which the atoms link together determines all of the particular characteristics of the substance they form. Most importantly, it also determines their chemical ability to react in a special way in the millions of reactions going on in our bodies at every single instant.

Although it seemed to Dr. Warburg that the fatty acid called butyric acid should provide the oxygen he reasoned was necessary to stop cancer metabolism, the arrangement of the energy charged electrons in that fatty acid did not provide enough power for the desired reaction to take place. Dr. Budwig determined that linseed oil, which contained an abundance of two special essential fatty acids would provide that distinctive force necessary to make Warburg's prediction come true - and she was right!

THE ESSENCE OF LIFE

The life processes of humans is greatly dependent on the role of light (predominantly sunlight) and its transformations into photons, electrons and pi-electrons. The availability of unsaturated fatty acids plays a major role in the transfer of electrons and therefore in the effect that respiratory enzymes and auto-oxidation have on maintaining or restoring normal metabolism. Let's take it step by step:

Photon energy is emitted by the sun. They are the incredibly tiny particles of energy that make up light. It is difficult to understand, but these photons are both energy waves and matter at the same time. The are part of the electromagnetic field, a force that is still not completely understood by science. The electrons that orbit every atom in the universe, which, of course includes our bodies, are actually made up of two photons. This explains why you so often hear that life comes from the energy of the sun. It is fascinating that many ancient cultures worshipped the sun as a God. Electrons absorb these photons through resonance (vibration). It is believed that vibration is the basic energy of everything. Because Einstein, amongst many others have proven that energy and matter are never actually destroyed but merely transformed from one form to the other, it becomes clear that everything is some type of vibration. This, for me, links science and religion. It brings together humankind, all the universe and everything in it.

Electrons absorb photons which increase their energy level. The electron can also emit photons. This process involves great energy and is involved in every change of substance. This is precisely the energy that Warburg was unable to attain in the use of butyric acid, but was obtained by Budwig in using **linolenic** and **linoleic** acids which were so readily available in linseed oil. These two unsaturated fatty acids composed of three pi-electrons (high-energy) double bonds between atoms of the compound. They possess the ability to transfer immense amounts of energy. This electron configuration is found in **linseeds, carotene, saffron and many other plant substances.** They play an important role in the functions of the cellular membranes of plants and animals (including humans) and can easily assimilate and transport **oxygen.** This process is called oxidation and is responsible for the breakdown of tissue and the detoxification of cellular waste products and poisons. It is also responsible for maintaining metabolic processes.

Intense heating and the addition of anti-oxidants to food is utilized to prevent its oxidation and destruction. This processing of food changes the nature of these compounds and destroys their ability to perform these vital functions. The processing, therefore, effectively preserves "dead" food. The vital energy and the benefit to human metabolism is lost. Without a knowledge of chemistry, Hippocrates by simple observation knew and therefore advised us to eat only natural foods. You would think that 2,500 years later, now that we have the scientific basis for following this advice, the medical profession would do so. The control exerted by the pharmaceutical industry on the philosophy and practice of medicine has created an army of individuals that are totally unaware that they hold an arrogant and ignorant position.

The brain and nervous system are mainly composed of unsaturated lipids (fats), especially those with the triple unsaturated bonds. Efficient and healthy brain function responds remarkably to the intake of the important unsaturated fats and should be included in the treatment of any disease. In building the bridge between fats and proteins, the lightest of all atoms, hydrogen, boosts up its energy level by absorbing photons and after the transfer of electrons on the protein side releases them. Sulphur containing proteins, found in all cell membranes, are the vitally important substances in this reaction. The entire process takes place in every life process including fertilization, cell division, genetic integrity and embryonic growth.

THE PROOF

Dr. Budwig proved the fundamental role of pi-electrons in this process in 1951. She delivered her paper at important medical meetings and published her findings in her book: "Komische Krafte gegen den Krebs". In using cis-linoleic acid, an **unsaturated** fatty acid, Dr. Budwig accomplished what Warburg failed to do with butyric acid. O. Meyerhof in his 1920 experiment, used linseed oil fatty acids to increase, a thousand-fold, the recovery of frog muscle from oxygen depletion. Sadly, he failed to mention this in the summation of his experiment and it did not receive appropriate recognition. In spite of the recognition of this important finding by such scientific notables as Albert Szent-Gyorgi and Fritz Popp in 1976 and 1977 and the preceding work of Dr. Budwig, the role of unsaturated fatty acids in the prevention and treatment of cancer has been suppressed.

The implications of these reactions explain many phenomena that physicians, particularly those who utilize natural remedies, have observed. The presence of this incredible source of electron and energy transfer provides an understanding of the electromagnetic fields demonstrated so dramatically in Kerlian photography. It clarifies the significant differences observed in the use of ozone or hydrogen peroxide instead of oxygen. Most of all, it should satisfy the sceptics in establishment medicine as to why natural therapies must, by their very nature, be superior to any artificial drug produced. The photon energy which produces electrons likewise is different when produced by man-made machines, than when produced by solar energy. It could only be brain-washing that has prevented intelligent individuals from recognizing that foods, being a combination of "living" chemicals, could be more effective and safer than the artificial and toxic products of the laboratory.

Radiation therapy is responsible for the development of mutations. It causes a disturbance of natural function as compared to the electrons of solar photon energy. One can easily understand that the exposure to the sun is a potential threat today, not from the sun itself, but from the changes we have brought about in our atmosphere and in our body chemistry. If we are deficient in normal unsaturated fatty acids, or worse, if we are contaminated by altered and poisonous fatty acids, how can we remain in a normal relationship with our universe?

I spent several days in Freudenstadt visiting Dr. Budwig and each evening I returned to my hotel with papers she gave me to read. In one of the papers, where she referred to the work of Szent-Gyorgi and Popp, it stated that they both mentioned growth regulation in the red field of light. That information was based on the work that Dr. Budwig had done involving her use of ruby laser (laser in the **red** spectrum of light) in the treatment of cancer and its relationship to the fatty acids. This especially interested me, because I had performed the world's first double-blind study on the use of low power helium neon and infrared laser, both in the red spectrum of light, which demonstrated definite therapeutic benefit in the treatment of arthritis of the hands. My paper was presented at the highly respected World Congress of Pain (1984) in Seattle, Washington. This carefully controlled scientific sudy, using an extremely safe level of laser light, similar to that used to read labels on products in millions of stores throughout the world, was repeated and confirmed by two fully accredited, well-known American universities. The FDA has not given the needed recognition to these studies that would make this therapy readily available and reimbursable by health insurance. This inexpensive, completely safe therapy would naturally pose a serious threat to the multi-billion dollar market in the potentially dangerous anti-inflammatory steroidal and non-steroidal drugs. These drugs comprise the largest, most profitable segment of drug sales.

As early as 1952, using the new revolutionary technique of paper chromatography while working at the Federal Institute for Fat Research in Germany, Dr. Budwig established the importance of unsaturated fatty acids in cancer patients. Her analysis and foresight has been proven to be correct i.e. the basic order of all growth processes are disturbed by the electrically neutralized foods and fats and; that the resonance of the red spectrum of light plays a specific role in the reactivation, storage and absorption of photons in the pi-electron system. Dr. Budwig is adamant in her belief that scientific evidence supports our ability to counter the progress towards entropy (chaos) ''with the anti-entropy factor from solar energy, through resonance phenomena as an anti-entropy factor of life''. In simple terms, we can prolong life much more than it is now.

During our visit together, Dr. Budwig asked if I would be kind enough to review her most recent, but as yet unpublished paper, ''Nature In Its Appearance in The Autoxydable System of Man. - An Interdisciplinary Approach.'' and suggest corrections in the English translation. In this paper she discusses in depth the application of quantum physics in the interaction between matter, electrons and electromagnetic fields and, in particular, their relationship with light. Her analysis also dealt with the quantum physics of the oxidative and transporting enzymes so vital in the metabolic role of fatty acids in the redox (oxidation-reduction) system. It would be improper for me to disclose the particulars of an unpublished paper. However, in our conversation she discussed one extremely important fact, of which I was not aware, I will pass it on to you just as I corrected and copied it from her paper. It is actually of public record, so I do not believe I am breaching a confidence. This information has been effectively ignored by the press, probably because they were not aware of its significance and its incredible impact on world health has been hidden from view.

THE UNHEEDED WARNING

IN 1977, THE WORLD HEALTH ORGANIZATION IN GENEVA, WITH AGREEMENT OF THE UNITED NATIONS AND THE FAO IN ROME, MADE THE FOLLOWING RECOMMENDATION:
IN THE LIGHT OF PRESENT KNOWLEDGE IT SEEMS PRUDENT TO RECOMMEND, FOR FUTURE LINES OF RESEARCH TO FOLLOW THESE REQUIREMENTS FOR EFA'S (LINOLEIC\LINOLENIC-FATTY ACID), THAT IT IS DESIRABLE THAT THEY ARE NOT LOST BY COMMERCIAL PROCESSING AND THAT THE PROBLEM MUST BE ADDRESSED BY LAW.

ANOTHER UNFILLABLE PREDICTION

When science proudly announces another discovery in the infinite chain of biological processes and suggests that we will soon have an artificial chemical answer to whatever disease they are investigating, they are naive in their understanding of the complexity of biological processes. The continued search for answers without understanding the role of photon energy and the electromagnetic fields and that the whole is significantly more than the sum of its parts, will reap only temporary or emergent relief and often a worse fate from the products born of such simplistic thinking. I had been able, in some instances, to accept the use of surgery and even some very limited use of radiation in the past, but the work of Dr. Budwig has awakened serious consideration to even further restrictions of their use. Establishment chemotherapy, in my view, represents a total abomination and should be discarded. The chemotherapy of the unsaturated fatty acids in the form of linseed oil makes more sense to me. After all, the "chemist" that made it is far more reliable than the ones who gave us thalidomide and the hundreds of other drugs which have been taken off the market because of their deadly effects.

MORE ABOUT LINSEED OIL -
ITS USES AND SUCCESSES

The hours spent reviewing the roles in body metabolism of linolenic and linoleic acid, the two fatty acids which linseed oil has in higher concentration than any other oil, helped me appreciate Dr. Budwig's monumental accomplishment. These two fatty acids are the essential ingredients in many vital body functions: they form prostaglandins which play a major role in the inflammatory response of the body to injury and disease; they effect the enzyme activity of the brain; the clotting mechanism of the blood as well as blood flow and blood pressure; repairs injury to the inside of the blood vessel walls; prevents the aggregation of platelets in the blood, thus reducing the formation of obstructing plaque (arteriosclerosis); effect favorably, risk factors in coronary heart disease; is significantly involved in the immune defenses, protects against auto immune disease, is found in sperm and in the retina of the eye.

Dr. Budwig related to me many clinical examples from her own experience, many of which her innumerable students have likewise reported in their own practices. The many physicians throughout the world who have used her approach for three decades confirm the success of her treatment in the following problems. Amongst those cited in our conversation and in her publications are:

✛ Cancer
✛ Arteriosclerosis
✛ Strokes
✛ Myocardial infarction (heart attack)
✛ Cardiac arrhythmias (irregular heart beat)
✛ Fatty degeneration of the liver
✛ Reduction of bronchospasm in the lungs
✛ Normalization of intestinal activity and function of the intestine
✛ Regulation of gastric secretion (stomach ulcers and hyperacidity)
✛ Prostatic hypertrophy (enlarged prostate)
✛ Reduction and repair of arthritic degeneration and inflammation

✛ Many dermatological problems (particularly eczema and psoriasis of the skin)

✛ Slows and improves many of the problems of aging and old age

✛ Improves brain function

✛ Beneficial in correcting diseases of immune deficiency and those believed to be a result of autoimmunity i.e. (multiple sclerosis, rheumatoid arthritis, etc.)

Sounds like an unbelievable panacea? Why not? Essential fatty acids are essential to life and the average diet is seriously deficient in them.

The books, articles, papers and conversation that Dr. Budwig made me privy to, as well as conversations with other physicians and friends of patients, provided many clinical stories from which I will recount a few (the names have been changed).

Timmy was diagnosed with Hodgkin's disease when he was only seven years old. He underwent surgery, followed by 24 treatments with radiation. He was then placed on additional therapies of an experimental nature. The experts subjected this child to painful and destructive therapies at immense cost, in the hope it would be of some help. Never was a cure even considered. When Timmy "failed to respond" to these "heroic" measures, he was declared incurable. Death was predicted in six months and he was then, mutilated and debilitated, sent home to die.

The parents, in desperation, searched the world for specialists trying to find an answer to their tragic situation. A prominent newspaper took up the cause and ran stories and editorials pleading for help for this doomed child. All the specialists that responded, agreed that the bitterly cruel prognosis was correct, the child would die. At this moment of dark despair and hopelessness, the family's prayers were answered. A miracle was in the making. The press printed the story. Timmy's mother had received an article from a friend about one of Dr. Budwig's speeches in which she had described her therapy for cancer. It gave the family the only hope they had in months. They contacted Dr. Budwig. For the first time in two years, after only five days on Dr. Budwig's program, Timmy's breathing returned to normal. He showed steady progress. His improvement was so remarkable that he was soon back in school and even took part in crafts and sports. Eleven years later, Timmy, at age eighteen, looked great and was doing very well in his university studies. He gives thanks daily for having been sent Dr. Johanna Budwig, the valiant woman to whom he owes his life.

Most specialists told Mary that the tumor under her eye would have to be removed surgically. The cancerous tumor was growing inside far more than the swelling that was visible on her face. There was bone involvement, and it had progressed to far for radiation to be effective. The surgery was to be extensive and would cause a major disfigurement of her face. She was young, and although she feared for her life, Mary could not bear the thought of being so horribly mutilated. Dr. Budwig's natural therapy came to her attention. She was extremely skeptical, but desperate as she was, she tried it. Within four months, the swelling had disappeared under her eye and tests were performed at the university hospital. One of the physicians said that if he had not had the previous records and x-rays, he would not believe that she had ever had a cancer. Her latest tests showed hardly any trace of residual tumor. She and her family are eternally grateful to Dr. Budwig and the natural formula which turned a gruesome prediction into a bright future.

In a relatively short period of time Sandy, had become paralyzed almost completely. His sight was severely impaired and he quickly lost control of his body functions. Tests revealed that he had a brain tumor that had caused arachnoidal bleeding, and that he was beyond help. He chose to die at home and was discharged from the hospital. A friend suggested that he give the Budwig formula a try. With nothing to lose, he started on the Budwig regimen. The paralysis receded, his eyesight improved and he was able to urinate naturally. Within a short period of time he was able to return to part-time work. His re-examination at the research center revealed that his reflexes had returned to normal. Ten years later, his examinations at the research center were still normal. Medical journals have recounted this incredible story of recovery and he has become the proverbial "text-book" case. No surgery, no radiation, no chemotherapy, just the simple diet that Dr. Budwig has fought to bring to the attention of the world.

The story of Dr. Siegfried Ernst is one that is very dramatic, and because he is a well-known colleague, I am devoting a separate section to him. It follows shortly.

Dr. Budwig's struggle to get linseed oil accepted, is only one example of the many non-patentable inexpensive and safe remedies for cancer and all the degenerative diseases, which comprise 90% of the cases in medicine, that offer significant improvement and even cures. Basic nutritional knowledge is vital in the prevention and cure of cancer and all disease. Has your doctor informed you, for example, that you can protect your family by changing the way you barbecue your meat. Do you know that the way you may doing it now, can be more dangerous than smoking thirty packs of cigarettes? I happened to hear it one time on television not too long ago. What if you missed it? What if you missed the information that appeared in one of the more than ten thousand journals printed each year? You wouldn't know where to look and your doctor doesn't have the time. He gets his "quick fix" from the pharmaceutical sales people or from journals that, almost always, print only articles reflecting the "drug philosophy".

Now for the story of Dr. Siegfried Ernst...

LUNCH WITH DR. SIEGFRIED ERNST

During one of my interviews with Dr. Johanna Budwig at her home in Freudenstadt, the phone rang and a happy and lively interview in German ensued. In a few minutes Dr. Budwig asked me to come to the phone.

"Take the phone," she said, "this is Dr. Ernst, the friend I told you about. Speak with him and confirm anything you would like."

Our conversation lasted approximately ten minutes and I tried to remember as much as I could. Most of the facts had already been related to me by Dr. Budwig. When I returned to my hotel I jotted down whatever I could recall. The next day was Friday and I was scheduled to leave in the morning for Stuttgart. My return flight was on Sunday at eight in the morning. Because it required a very early wake-up and I did not want to risk missing it, I decided to arrive there a day early. After purchasing as many of Dr. Budwig's books as possible at a local apothecary, I took a taxi to the train station and was on my way. The plane that I had hoped to take was full, and I was advised that I would be able to get a flight out of Munich. On the way to Munich the train stopped at Ulm, which in our phone conversation, Dr. Ernst had mentioned was his home. I decided to get off the train and try to find him. Within an hour I had a hotel room and arranged to meet with Dr. Ernst the following morning.

I spent the day with Dr. Ernst who, though in his late seventies, seemed tireless. This is a rare dedicated man in every possible way. He is devoted to family, church, city and humanity. He counted amongst his personal friends the present Pope and many other dignitaries. Although he is undoubtedly grateful to Dr. Budwig, he disagreed on various points with reference to her therapy being complete. He felt as I do, that if there is a large tumor, it should be removed without mutilation or incapacitation to the patient. The reason being its tremendous toxic effect, and thus incredible drain on our protective resources. I must remind you that Dr. Budwig is a purist with reference to the efficacy of her own therapy. She firmly believes that any failures are caused by non-compliance on the part of the patient or alterations in the protocol on the part of the physician. Although she may be correct, I prefer to use every possible safe and non-destructive technique on behalf of the patient against such a formidable enemy as cancer. I would happily change my mind if comparative studies were available. In early tumors, her therapy should be sufficient. It becomes a judgement call in referrence to surgery, but I personally reject chemotherapy or radiation almost without exception.

Dr. Ernst related in detail many fascinating episodes of his life. For this book, I will relate only the cancer story. He told me that seventeen years ago he had developed a cancer of the stomach for which he had major surgery. It had required removal of his stomach and left him with a great number of digestive problems and considerable debilitation. His professional life had virtually come to an end. He was approximately sixty years old at the time. He had great difficulty in continuing to practice medicine.

Two years later he had a recurrence of the cancer and was offered chemotherapy as the only available remedy. There was little hope for survival, and knowing that chemotherapy was not only ineffectual, but completely destructive of the quality of life, he refused. It was then that he turned to Dr. Budwig for help. For two years he religiously followed the dietary routine outlined in this book and , in addition, he used the application of the linseed oil to his body every evening. The oil was applied to the abdominal area and wrapped with cloth bandages. He has since persisted in remaining true to the diet 95% of the time and continues the low fat cottage cheese and linseed oil daily. It has been fifteen years since the recurrence of the stomach cancer and the institution of the Budwig therapy. Dr. Ernst has had good quality of life except for relatively minor problems with eating and digesting food. The simple addition of digestive enzymes and other supplements have made his existence almost completely normal.

Virtually all individuals with a recurrence of this type of cancer rarely last a year. If they agree to chemotherapy, the time gained is negligible, and the side-effects from the chemotherapy makes it regrettable. Of course the establishment will dismiss the results as a "spontaneous remission" in spite of the fact that it is unheard of, except when patients go for simple alternative therapies. I seriously think that alternative (orthodox) physicians should create a specialists' designation and advertise themselves as "practice limited to spontaneous remissions". If a colleague attributed Dr. Ernst's results to happenstance, I am sure Ernst would answer in the polite German equivalent of "Why don't you come off it!"

Dr. Ernst's son, Martin, also a physician, joined us in the afternoon for several hours. I was saddened to find out that the physicians in Germany faced many of the same problems as doctors in the United States. I listened to the cases of physicians who brought their family members for successful non-establishment treatments, but renounced and refused those same remedies to their patients. I was angered at one story about a physician who had treated a child with leukemia with non-toxic natural remedies, who was brought to court by the medical establishment. The parents had refused chemotherapy from another doctor and had requested the alternative therapy from the doctor who was now being charged with depriving the child with proper medical treatment. The child survived the same amount of time she would have on chemotherapy, without any of the debilitating, painful and dehumanizing effects.

Establishment medicine, with little or no evidence to support their barbaric use of these highly toxic drugs, continue to make fortunes while their patients spend their last days vomiting, debilitated baldheaded and without dignity. While patients suffer from "cutting edge" therapy, the physician places his head comfortably on his pillow at night, content that he has served humanity with the best "anyone" has to offer. His dreams and his waking hours know nothing of the other world out there that has existed for five thousand years. Besides, how dare anyone suggest that a tribal medicine man or a dissident colleague could accomplish more. It is incredible to me that physicians could accept the fact that a single artificial chemical compound created in a laboratory could cure or control a disease and reject the idea that a natural food, with its many chemical compounds, could do the same or infinitely better.

Our conversation lasted for many hours and he confirmed much of what Dr. Budwig had told me and more. I recalled the many stories of patients she had treated. I had been made privy to her private papers. She carefully guarded the identity of her patients and I respected her, all the more, for it. My conversation with the incredibly kind and sensitive Dr. Ernst recanted some of the information and results I had learned in my visit with Dr. Budwig. I must admit that whatever skepticism I may have had, when Dr. Budwig was emphatic that her diet actually prevented and cured cancer, disappeared after my memorable meeting with Dr. Ernst. He was both a colleague and a fellow cancer victim who had been truly cured, not just a five-year survival.

****

THE BUDWIG THERAPY

BUDWIG DIET

As incredible and simple as it may seem, it is true - the cornerstone of the Budwig treatment is **low fat cottage cheese and cold pressed, unprocessed linseed oil!** But don't stop here and run to the store. There is more and it is important that you be completely informed if you want the best results. Of course, any improvement in diet is beneficial, but if you are dealing with cancer "any improvement" is not good enough.

The diet is presented in two parts. The first section, I. PREVENTING CANCER, is for individuals who do not have cancer, but who understand that the diets they have been eating all their lives are a definite cause of most cancers. This diet is designed to correct much of the damage which has undoubtedly occurred. The second section, II. IF YOU HAVE CANCER, is for individuals diagnosed with cancer and are in need of a more aggressive approach. FOLLOW IT TO THE LETTER!

I. PREVENTING CANCER

THE BASIC MIXTURE:

PURE VIRGIN COLD-PRESSED UNPROCESSED
LINSEED OIL (FLAXSEED OIL) - - - - 1 TABLESPOON
LOW FAT COTTAGE CHEESE - - - - - -1/2 to 1 CUP

This basic combination of fatty acids and sulfur rich protein can be taken alone or in combination as a mixture. However, there are many ways that it can be varied by adding flavoring or other food ingredients to suit your own taste. (see below)

THE RECOMMENDED DIET

The diet which is slowly being recognized by all medical authorities as a cancer preventive, stresses the intake of:

FRESH FRUITS - - - - - - - -3 to 4 MEDIUM SIZE
PORTIONS DAILY.

FRESH VEGETABLES - - - - -4 to 6 CUPS (SEVERAL

TABLESPOONS OF LINSEEDS AND/OR 1 TO 2 TABLESPOONS OF THE OIL CAN BE USED IN THE SALAD DRESSING OR ON THE VEGETABLES, BE SURE TO INCLUDE CABBAGE, BROCCOLI, AND MAITAKE MUSHROOMS.

UNPROCESSED WHOLE GRAIN BREADS AND CEREALS - - - - - - - - -3 to 4 CUPS OR PORTIONS.

FRESH FISH (PREFERABLY COLD WATER VARIETY) - - - - - - - - - - - 4 to 8 oz. An excellent source of the omega-3 fatty acids is rainbow trout.

FRESH MEAT - BRED WITHOUT HORMONES, FAT PRODUCING DIETS OR FEED THAT HAS BEEN GROWN WITH PESTICIDES OR ANTIBIOTICS......3oz. TWO TO THREE TIMES A WEEK.

LIQUIDS - BOTTLED WATER. IF POSSIBLE IT SHOULD BE PURIFIED BY REVERSE OSMOSIS, DISTILLATION AND OZONATION. THERE ARE MANY INDIVIDUALS WHO HAVE DIFFICULTY WITH DRINKING THE EIGHT GLASSES A DAY THAT IS RECOMMENDED. SUGGESTION; PLACE ONE GLASS OF YOUR FAVORITE JUICE IN A LITER OR QUART BOTTLE AND FILL THE REMAINDER WITH WATER. IT IS REFRESHING.

**DON'T FORGET -
HERBAL TEAS - ESSAIC FORMULA,
CHAPARRAL, ETC.**

FRESH FRUIT JUICES (CITRUS FRUITS SHOULD NOT BE TAKEN WITHIN SEVERAL HOURS OF THE LINSEED OIL - COTTAGE CHEESE PORTIONS)

CAUTION: REMEMBER THAT EATING ANY PROCESSED OILS WILL COUNTERACT EVERYTHING YOU ARE TRYING TO DO. THEY ARE POISON, AS ARE ALL FRIED FOODS. ELIMINATE AS MUCH SUGAR AS POSSIBLE

FROM THE DIET. REMEMBER THAT HONEY (NOT ROYAL JELLY) IS PRIMARILY SUGAR. PREPARED FOODS MUST BE DEVOID OF ALL ARTIFICIAL PRESERVATIVES OR CHEMICAL ADDITIVES. ARTIFICIAL SWEETENERS ARE ABSOLUTELY FORBIDDEN! IF GOD DIDN'T MAKE IT OR YOU CAN'T PRONOUNCE IT - DON'T EAT IT!

HELPFUL HINTS:

The first time I tried linseed oil on a salad, I was pleasantly surprised. I had expected it to taste strange or unusual. It didn't - IT TASTED GREAT! The mixture with the low fat cottage cheese was even more exciting than I anticipated. I actually looked forward to eating a slice of the multi-grain bread covered with a thick layer of the mixture. I do realize that you cannot argue taste, and that taste varies tremendously. With that in mind, I am providing a whole list of ingredients and suggestions for ways of making the Budwig "formula" a delight for your palate.

For Breakfast:

Fruit Juice

Cereal - ground linseeds, whole grains and nuts raisins
chopped fresh fruits linseed oil and low-fat
cottage cheese, 1/3 to 1/2 cup low-fat milk, and
honey mixed well in a blender

Eggs - blend 2 eggs with 1 teaspoon of linseed oil and
1 tablespoon low-fat cottage cheese - add
chopped tomato, onions and green pepper, herbs
and spices - slowly bake or broil

"Coffee" - made from roasted cereals

For Lunch or Dinner:

Salad - any desired mixture of greens, vegetables or fruits.

Dressings: low-fat cottage cheese and linseed oil mixture, then add the ingredients for the followingdressings:

Honey Mustard: 1 tsp. honey and 1/2 tsp. of Dijon mustard

Creamy Italian: vinegar, herbs (Italian), then for taste variation, add any combination of spices, mustard, raw egg, garlic, onion powder, crushedanchovies

Green Goddess: minced spinach, cucumber parsley, lemon and dill.

Mexican: minced chile, red peppers,tomato onion, herbs and spices.

Fruit: honey,crushed nuts, poppy seeds and linseeds - touchof cinnamon, lemon and/or mustard if desired.

SOUPS:

Gazpacho Soup: dilute basic mixture with low-fat milk and add: tomatos, garlic, cucumber, onions, herbs and spices-blend well and chill.

Bean Soups: prepare your favorite soup in the usual way and add the Budwig mix to it.

Other Soups: tomato and onion soups can be made as usual and the Budwig mix added.

COOKED VEGETABLES: lightly steam, cook and then coat with linseed oil and spices. Honey and oil isgreat for corn and sweet potato. Baked potatogoes well with mix, oil alone or with onions,parsley etc.

Desert: The basic mixture plus; cut-up peaches, berries, flavoring, nuts, cinnamon, cloves, nutmeg, honey and your personal creativeness.

II. IF YOU HAVE CANCER:

IT IS IMPERATIVE THAT YOU FOLLOW THE DIET EXACTLY - NO CHEATING IS ALLOWED! DR. BUDWIG PLACED GREAT STRESS ON FOLLOWING THE DIET EXACTLY. HER MANY YEARS OF EXPERIENCE HAS CONVINCED HER THAT FAILURES DO NOT OCCUR EXCEPT WHEN THE PATIENT IS LAX WITH HER TREATMENT. USE THE LINSEED OIL MORE FREQUENTLY DURING AND FOR IN-BETWEEN MEAL SNACKS.

WRAPPING THE BODY IN LINSEED OIL SOAKED CLOTHS, THE PART THAT IS EFFECTED WITH CANCER, IS VERY HELPFUL. FOR EXAMPLE, IF YOU HAVE A LIVER CANCER, WRAP THE WAIST. IF IT IS THE LUNGS, WRAP THE CHEST. IF IT IS THE BRAIN, WRAP THE HEAD AND NECK, AND SO ON. THIS IS BEST ACCOMPLISHED DURING THE NIGHT AND WHENEVER THE OPPORTUNITY ALLOWS. THE OIL CAN BE MIXED WITH ROSE WATER TO ADD AN ESTHETIC TOUCH. COLD PRESSED AND UNPROCESSED WALNUT, PUMPKIN AND SOYBEAN OIL, CAN BE USED IN ADDITION TO LINSEED OIL FOR VARIETY. I STRONGLY RECOMMEND, IN ADDITION TO THE VITAMINS AND MINERALS ALREADY SUGGESTED, THAT PARTICULAR EMPHASIS BE PLACED ON MAKING SURE YOU TAKE THE RECOMMENDED DOSES OF VITAMIN C, E, SELENIUM AND BETA-CAROTENE.

****

IMPORTANT:

SEE THE SECTION ON SPECIFIC CANCER THERAPIES FOR A TOTAL THERAPEUTIC APPROACH.

Chapter 6

Nature's Food Medicines

GARLIC

Garlic has, for five thousand years, been used as a medicinal food. It is truly a natural antibiotic and anti-parasitic. Almost every civilization has recognized its medical use. It contains many vitamins and minerals, as well as amino acids and sulphur compounds. Doctors of natural medicine have long used garlic for problems of **high blood pressure, cholesterol and diabetes.** In 1990, the first World Congress, devoted solely to the health significance of garlic and garlic constituents, was held in Washington, D.C.

T. H. Abdullah, in the journal of the National Medical Association, 1988, discussed the wide application of garlic.

Garlic has been used in **viral infections, fungus infections and as an anti-cancer agent** (E. Fujita, Cell Biol Toxicol, 1986).

Studies have shown that garlic **protects against radiation damage** (R. Lin, 1990) and as an **anti-carcinogenic** (J. Milner and J. Liu, 1990).

S. Hoon, et al., also presented a paper at the World Congress which showed that garlic was **more effective against melanoma than synthetic drugs.**

A study by Dr. Mei Xing of the Shandong Medical College in China, in 1981, demonstrated that garlic reduced the levels of nitrite in the blood within four hours after ingestion.

Many studies indicate that it is beneficial in the treatment and prevention of high blood pressure, diabetes, heart disease, pneumonia, dysentery and yeast infections. It is generally considered to be an immune stimulant. The popularity of garlic amongst health food adherents, has produced many reference books, some of which are completely devoted to garlic alone.

****

GREEN TEA

If you have ever eaten in a Japanese restaurant, the delicate pale green tea is actually a source of **anti-carcinogenic** substances.

Epigallocatechin Gallate (EGCG) found in green tea, is a chemical which inhibits the growth of cancers and lowers cholesterol (T. Chisaka, et al., Chem Pharm Bull. Tokyo 1988). EGCG appears to work as a scavenger of free radicals and neutralizes active substances which alter DNA, which thus cause carcinogenic changes. EGCG fed to mice inhibited the development of cancer of the **lung** and **liver cancers**. This remarkable finding was reported in 1991 at the Fourth Chemical Congress of North America.

The application of this substance to the skin also acts as a cancer preventative and works for tumors of the gastrointestinal tract (Y. Fugita, Japanese Journal of Cancer Research, 1989, H. Fujiki, Basic Life Sciences, 1990). It has been recommended as a daily cancer preventative and is extremely inexpensive.

Rutgers University scientists have confirmed that cancers of the **stomach** and **lung** can be prevented by as much as 60% in laboratory mice.

D. Mourlatos and his group noted that another substance in the tea, theophylline, works synergistically with the anti-cancer drug, Chlorambucil and increased its chemical activity.

H.U. Gali in Cancer Research, 1991 and Carcinogenesis, 1992, reported on another ingredient, tannic acid, which appears to be effective topically and internally against cancer.

****

DMSO

Dimethyl sulfoxide (DMSO) is found in vegetables, fruits, grains and milk. It is also a normal chemical in the human body. Commercially, it is used as a solvent and obtained from wood, coal and oil. It is used in medicine around the world, but typically, in the United States the FDA limits its use to interstitial cystitis of the bladder. The restriction by the FDA was placed because there was some question about "possible" harmful changes occurring in the eyes of test animals. However, not one single documented case of eye damage in humans, has been demonstrated in over 25 years. Because it is extremely inexpensive and unpatentable, it is not likely that extensive investigation, which costs millions, will ever be done.

NOTE: DMSO is an incredible chemical, which markedly facilitates the transport and absorption of other substances. (L. Stjernval, 1969, E. J. Tucker, 1968 and C. A. Thuning, 1983). **It is extremely important in bringing anticarcinogenic therapies to the site of the cancer.**

It has been found that DMSO will normalize **leukemia** cells (H. Sugano, 1975).

DMSO does not kill cancer cells, but appears to reverse their abnormal characteristics. By using DMSO in **conjunction with cancer chemotherapy,** the chemotherapy dose can be reduced, while maintaining its effect and, thereby, also reduces the toxicity involved (R.F. Pommier, An J Surg. 1988).

C. B. Gerharz, et al., in the British Journal of Cancer 1989, confirmed the use of DMSO in combination with other substances in significantly improving the anti-cancer effect.

This same finding applies to **prostate cancer,** when it is used in conjunction with 5-FU (D. D. Nickey, et al., Prostate, 1989).

In my own investigations, I have found that most cancer clinics providing alternative therapies, use intravenous DMSO in conjunction with the daily treatments involving Laetrile, Vitamin C, etc.. DMSO has only one side effect of which I am aware, i.e. all patients have a characteristic garlic-like odor from their body when receiving DMSO.

75

ENZYME THERAPY

Enzymes are manufactured in the body from amino acids. They are also obtained from the foods that we eat. Life could not exist without enzymes. What role do they play in the life process? They:

✛ Digest all the food we eat making it small enough to pass through the pores of the intestine into the blood.

✛ Rebuild and repair muscle, nerve, bone and glandular tissue.

✛ Assist in storing excess food in the liver and muscles.

✛ Fix iron in the blood cells.

✛ Assist in the coagulation of blood.

✛ Decompose hydrogen peroxide and liberate oxygen.

✛ Promotes oxidation.

✛ Converts waste products of metabolisminto urea and uric acid for elimination.

✛ Converts protein into fat or sugar.

✛ Converts fats into carbohydrate Converts carbohydrate into fat.

✛ Converts all starches and sugars into dextrose.

✛ Converts dextrose into glycogen for storage.

✛ Assists in the burning of fats and glycogen into energy.

However, the enzymes in all foods are completely destroyed when cooked, baked, roasted, stewed, broiled, boiled or fried.

Historically, plant enzymes (i.e. Papain, from Papaya fruit) have been used to treat skin tumors. Pancreatic enzymes gained popularity because of the work done by Dr. John Beard and continued by Dr. Ernst T. Krebs, Jr., in the treatment of cancer.

Dr. Andrew Weil who has written extensively on natural medicine, does not feel that enzymes are useful because they are destroyed in the intestinal tract (He does, however, recommend pancreatic and stomach enzymes for digestive problems.) I have to respectfully disagree with Dr. Weil. In arguing this point, Peter R. Rothschild, MD, PhD, stated in Enzyme Therapy - In Immune Complex and Free Radical Contingent Diseases (University Labs Press, 1988),

" ... serum levels of the enzymes increased remarkably in vivo (in the human) after oral applications."

To those who argue that this could be due to enzymogens in the serum, he replies,

" ... if ... we admit the possibility of enzymogenic activation, the fact remains unchanged, since such activation occured without exception only after ingestion of the enzyme. ... (if) something that acted as a co-factor to activate the enzymogens, (it) necessarily had to be absorbed in the intestines. By sheer logic, it is obvious that ... (it) had to be furnished by the ingested enzymes."

Rothschild, is a full professor at the National Autonomous University in Mexico, with doctorates in Medicine and Biochemistry and a masters in Quantum Physics. He was nominated for the Nobel Prize in Quantum Physics. He goes on to explain that his experiments have demonstrated **that enzymes do, in fact, pass through the mucous and submucous layers in the intestines.** By emulsification, they are turned into liposomes that traverse even the muscle layers, reach the lymphatics and hence to the superior vena cava where they bypass the liver and are then transported to all the tissues of the body via the blood circulation.

****

DIGESTIVE ENZYMES

The digestive Enzymes comprise only a small number of the enzymes produced and utilized by the body. Protease, Amylase, Lipase, Trypsin and Chymotrypsin are the primary digestive enzymes. Adequate production is necessary for the breakdown, absorption and utilization of our food. Experiments have shown that without this process successfully taking place minute globules of food matter can traverse the intestinal wall and create serious disturbances in metabolism resulting in disease.

****

ONCONASE

This enzyme-like protein is obtained from a common frog

(Rana pipiens). It is similar to ribonuclease, a pancreatic enzyme. S. M. Mikulski, in the Journal of the National Cancer Institute, 1990, demonstrated its anti-cancer effect in a specific carcinoma in laboratory mice with dramatic results. Actual cures were obtained and longevity was increased markedly. Laboratory studies on rats and dogs produced side effects which diminished when the dosage was decreased. The original work performed by W. Ardelt and reported in the Journal of Biochemistry, 1991, is currently undergoing FDA approved trials for various types of cancer. There are indications that this drug may be effective in pancreatic, colorectal, esophageal and lung cancers (J. J. Costanzi, ASCO, Abs.#268).

****

ENZYME PREPARATIONS

Wobe Mugos produced, in Germany, from papaya thymus, pancreas, lentils and peas, is a widely used preparation amongst alternative therapeutic physicians. I mention it by name because it is the only preparation in Europe I know of (there probably are others).

There is evidence that enzymes can increase T-cell counts (P.B. Holland, et al., British Journal of Cancer, 1975, and F. W. Bube, Folia Haematologie, 1981).

Many physicians I have talked to, feel that the use of enzyme preparations, such as Wobe Mugos, improve the effectiveness of their therapies. The belief is that it breaks down the mucous-membranous wall of tumor cells thus permitting greater accessibility to therapeutic agents.

There are many excellent products manufactured in the U.S.A. A complete listing of sources can be found in the resource section of this book.

****

Chapter 7

Vital Vittles - Vitamins And Minerals

VITAMINS

For many decades, establishment medicine has branded as "quacks", those practitioners of medicine, chiropractic, naturopathy, homeopathy and nutrition, who advocate the use of vitamins, minerals and a host of natural supplements for the treatment of disease and the maintenance of health. Medical physicians, for the most part, ignore the advice given by the "Father of Medicine" and the originator of the oath that they take. Hippocrates, in the fifth century B.C., proclaimed, **"Let your food be your medicine and let your medicine be your food."** Modern medical establishment scientists look upon vitamins as merely a fact of life and something which, when deficient in the body, causes disease. It is only in recent years that certain vitamins have been recognized as preventives of disease, including cancer. That section of the public which has advocated and followed a program of healthy foods as a means of staying well and even treating disease, have been disdainfully referred to as "faddists". The leaders of the health food movement have long advocated the daily intake of mostly vegetables and fruit. In the last few years, scientists have proven that vegetables and fruit juices have anti-cancer actions, i.e. keep the cells from developing mutations that produce cancer cells. In 1990, R. Edenharder and his associates proved that vegetables and fruits can inhibit mutations in cells in the laboratory. The vegetables which exhibited the strongest anti-mutation activity were cabbage (red), asparagus, broccoli, carrots, lettuce, celery and green peppers. My goodness, has the establishment gone "faddist"?

VITAMIN A

Vitamin A is extremely important for immunity and works to protect the thymus gland which produces the hormone that is essential in helping us fight against infectious agents and carcinogens. It also works to detoxify poisons, either produced in the body or that are introduced from outside the body. Vitamin A is an anti-oxidant which means that it destroys the chemicals produced by the body during its metabolism which are meant for waste disposal. However, during the period of time which elapses between their production and their excretion, they can be extremely dangerous unless they are neutralized and this is performed by the anti-oxidants, of which Vitamin A is one of the most important. Vitamin A also plays an important role in the formation of protein, for the growth process and in the chemical processes that allow us to see at night. Shortly after its discovery in 1922, Vitamin A was found to be effective in the prevention of cancer. However, this was largely ignored. From countries all over the world scientists have reaffirmed the role of Vitamin A in the treatment and prevention of cancer. Studies on laboratory animals have repeatedly shown that it can protect laboratory animals from cancer of the gastro-intestinal track, lungs, stomach and the uterus. These articles now number in the thousands.

Blood levels of Vitamin A were found to be much lower in men who developed cancer of the prostate. The National Cancer Institute studied 2,500 men over the age of fifty for a period of ten years. The risk of developing prostate cancer was directly proportional to the low level of Vitamin A in the blood serum. In 1974, the National Cancer Institute did its largest study and again found that the level of Vitamin A had a direct bearing on the development of prostate cancer. The lower the level of Vitamin A, the higher the instance of prostate cancer.

In the European Journal of Epidemiology in 1990, French

scientists headed by J. Dardingus and his associates, studied the risks of lung cancer and the intake of Vitamin A and Beta-Carotene. The work included experimental animals as well as humans. Once again, a direct correlation was made between the intake of Vitamin A and Beta-Carotene and the development of this dreaded tumor. It was found that Beta-Carotene was a preventative and Vitamin A was effective as a treatment for lung cancer.

Summary: Supplementation of Vitamin A should be held below 50,000 international units per day. The presence of Vitamin A and Beta-carotene in the diet reduces the risk of pre-cancerous lesions of the cervix. A diet rich in beta-carotene lowers the risk of developing stomach, lung, oral, larynx and esophageal cancers.

****

BETA-CAROTENE

The preventive action of beta-carotene on cancer of the lung is more powerful than vitamin A. Once again the electrical charge present in the compound appears to play an important role. Electromagnetic forces are discussed elsewhere in greater detail. Beta-carotene destroys the layer of mucous which coats and protects the cancer cell from attack by the immune system. **Studies indicate that as much as an 80 % reduction in the rate of bronchial and lung cancer can be achieved by regularly eating carrots in our diets. There also appears to be a reduction of cancer of the colon by as much as 55 %.**

At the Albert Einstein College of Medicine in New York City, laboratory animals fed beta-carotine more than 30 days after exposure to cancer causing chemicals did not develop the number of tumors that were expected to occur.

Beta-carotine was protective against both late and early stages of tumor development and growth. Dr. Seifter who carried out this research recommended five to ten mg of beta-carotine for basic protection and twice that amount for smokers.

A study done by P.R. Palan at the Albert Einstein College of Medicine in New York City studied the levels of beta-carotine in the tissues of cervical, endometrial, ovarian, breast, colon, lung, liver and rectal cancers. In all of these tissues the levels of beta-carotene was lower than in the surrounding normal tissues.

A similar finding was noted in breast cancer patients in the 1990 National Cancer Institute Study done by N. Potischman and reported in the American Journal of Clinical Nutrition. As one might expect no solid studies have been done on the role of high doses of beta-carotene in the treatment of human cancer. This, of course, represents the results of the profit motive, because beta-carotene cannot be patented.

Beta-carotene has been tested for treatment of a precancerous lesion of the mouth called leukoplakia. This study showed dramatic results with no toxicity in the treatment of these oral lesions. It was felt that beta-carotene would be an excellent candidate as a preventive agent in oral cancers. This study was performed by H.S. Garewal and Associates and reported in the Journal of Clinical Oncology in 1990. Experiments in laboratory mice have also revealed encouraging results. A particular type of sarcoma caused by a virus was injected into the mice. The administration of beta-carotene caused a regression of the tumors.

It was also noted that the beta-carotene protects the thymus gland which is a major part of our immune defense system. E. Seifter and his group reported this finding in the Journal of the National Cancer Institute in 1982. He expressed the definite opinion that the protective action on the Thymus gland was probably a significant factor in the anti-tumor activity.

E. R. Abril and his associates studied the effects of beta-carotene in laboratory blood of 6 human cancers. Their results indicated that beta-carotene stimulated the production of cytokines which are powerful substances which the body produces in fighting cancers and boosting immunity. Other studies by Garewal and W.F. Malone reported in the American Journal of Clinical Nutrition in 1991 that beta-carotene might be useful in preventing recurrences of tumors in individuals at great risk especially in the **upper gastro-intestinal tract.**

L.A. and A.B. Santamaria reported in Medical Oncological Tumor Therapie in 1990, that beta-carotene increased the disease-free interval between the initial occurrence of tumors of the **lung, breast, colon, urinary bladder and head and neck** cancers, and their recurrences.

A study was done in China with relation to liver cancer mortality and certain aspects of diet. The incidence of liver cancer was found to be high when there was an increased consumption of alcohol, rapeseed oil and mouldy corn. It was also noted that previous infections with hepatitis B seemed to contribute to an increase in the death rate occurrence from liver cancer. The study, however, was not able to link beta-carotene or vitamin and mineral consumption with the deaths. This study was published in the International Journal of Epidemiology in 1991 by A. W. Hsing.

E.R. Greenberg also did a study which showed that beta-carotene over a five year period reduced the reoccurrence rate of skin cancers unrelated to **melanoma**.

****

B-COMPLEX VITAMINS

Supplementation with B vitamins are extremely important with reference to immune system function and repair. Studies have been done which indicate that **cancer chemotherapy** causes deficiencies of many of the B Vitamins, particularly niacin, folic acid, B1, B2 and vitamin K. These findings were noted Postgraduate Medicine, 1990 by S. Dreisen et al. Whole grains, vegetables, liver, kidney, lean meats and halibut provide vitamin B in substantial amounts.

****

PYRIDOXINE

Pyridoxine (B6), was studied by G. Litwack at the Fels Research Institute, Temple University, Philadelphia, Pennsylvania. Studies with laboratory rats that had **liver** cancer revealed that B6 actually kills cancer cells. No affect was seen, however, on human cancer cells. They concluded that B6 was promising as a anti-cancer agent. It is my opinion that these scientists commit a grave error in using single vitamins in testing them against tumors. Elementary understanding should tell them that it takes a complete complement of all of the necessary vitamins and minerals to achieve a proper balance and effect in combating cancer cells. The individual studies done on specific vitamins certainly point to specific cancers in which they may play a role, however, it does not give a true picture of what actually happens in the body where so many other factors are necessary. It has been noted that a vitamin B6 deficiency has an adverse affect on the formation of DNA and the development of anti-bodies.

The role of vitamin B6 in genetics is of great significance because the development of cancer begins with the alteration of the genetic structure of cells. C.D. Simone and his group wrote about the immune effects of vitamin B6 in their article "Vitamins and Immunity" published in Acta Vitaminol Enzymology in 1982.

The Russian scientist V. Draudin-Krylenko, demonstrated that the formation of lung cancers in experimental animals could be stopped by injections of vitamin B6.

****

RIBOFLAVIN

Riboflavin was studied extensively by researchers at the Cancer Institute of the Chinese Academy of Medicine in Beijing in 1988. Vitamin B2 (Riboflavin) and Chinese herbal preparations proved to be dramatically effective in reducing the incidence of esophageal cancers.

****

FOLIC ACID

Folic acid which has played a major role in the treatment of certain types of anemia has also been noted to have a strong **anti-cancer** effect. Folic acid, which is found predominantly in dark green leafy vegetables, along with vitamin B12 was found to be helpful in the repair of lung tissue and in **preventing lung cancer** in smokers. Once again the role of vitamins in the formation of DNA is supported by scientists at the University of

Alabama Medical Center, who noted a reduction in carcinogenic changes in the lungs of smokers. This is another example where combinations, in this case folate, B12 and beta-carotene obviously has a protective affect. As usual, the Journal of the American Medical Association cautioned against the use of large doses B12 and folic acid (JAMA, 1988, D.C. Heimberger). The study they were referring to involved the use of **10 mg of folic acid and 500 mg of vitamin B12**. Yet, I know of no study that indicates that these doses are excessive or hold any danger of toxicity.

Another study in the Journal of the American Medical Association by C. Butterworth showed an association between folate deficiency and cervical dysplasia. Cervical dysplasia is often referred to as the precursor to the development of **cancer of the cervix**, which is the most common cancer amongst women in the world. Its incidence is highest in third world countries. The human papilloma virus, which is known to cause cervical cancer has also been related to low folate levels.

Butterworth also reported, that in an ongoing study he was conducting at the University of Alabama using 10mg of folic acid daily, there were no adverse side effects and positive cervical pap smears were reverting to normal.

In case there is any doubt that folate can be used to treat these early carcinogenic changes of the cervix, a study by J. Ran, published in Blood, 1990, revealed that cervical cells cleared up with the administration of folate.

I. Eto and C. Krumdieck, in the Journal of Advanced Experimental Medical Biology, 1986, expressed the view that the lack of folate may not in itself be cancer-causing, but certainly a deficiency renders an individual more susceptible to carcinogenic agents.

****

NICOTINAMIDE

The B vitamin Nicotinamide has been shown by M.R. Horsman to greatly **enhance** the cancericidal affect of the **chemotherapeutic agent** L-PAM. This was published in the British Journal of Cancer in 1986. A similar enhancing action was noted along with Cis-platin, another chemotherapeutic agent. Nicotinamide alone exhibits a preventive effect with relation to cancer but no evidence of anti-carcinogenic ability. These findings were noted by G. Chan and Q.C. Pan in Cancer Chemotherapeutic Pharmacology 1988.

An aspirin and nicotinic acid given before and after gama-ray radiation therapy resulted in a marked reduction in relapse of **bladder cancer** with an almost 300 % increase in the 5 years survival of these patients. This indicates an increase in resistance to tumors and was reported by A. I. Popow in the Russian Journal Medical Radiology in 1987.

****

CARNITINE

Carnitine, even though it can be manufactured by the body, is often referred to as **vitamin B-t**. However it does require the presence of two amino acids, several vitamins and minerals. M. Giovannini in the Journal of International Medical Research in 1991, indicated that carnitine is essential in pregnancy, breast feeding and infancy. Carnitine is extremely important and essential for the transport and oxidation of fatty acids which is discussed at length in another section of the book under linseed oil. The energy metabolism of cells is highly dependant on carnitine. It also appears that carnitine plays a role in the effect of the thymus hormone on the metabolism of cells and their ability to multiply. This is particularly important in reference to our white blood cells which are our first line of defense in infections and **cancer**. Older individuals are virtually devoid of thymus hormone and the use of carnitine seems to improve the ability of white cells to multiply in this group.

C. Franceschi, in the International Journal of Clinical Pharmacological Research, 1990 demonstrated that carnitine protected the white blood cells of older individuals from exposure to free radicals.

D. S. Sachan and W.L. Dodson, in the Journal of the American College of Nutrition in 1987, gave evidence that carnitine was destroyed by chemotherapy and resulted in a marked loss of energy.

C. De Simone in 1982, in Acta Vitaminol Enzymology and in another article published in German in the journal Arzneimittelforschung, also in 1982, wrote that the damage certain fats have on the immune system can be counteracted to a significant degree by carnitine.

When **carnitine** is added to the use of **Azelaic acid** in the treatment of **malignant melanoma**, it greatly enhances the transport of Azelaic acid into the cancer cell and thus facilitates its killing ability. Carnitine therefore should be useful in reducing the strength of Azelaic acid needed to be cancericidal. This opinion was voiced by B.J. Ward in the Journal of Investigative Dermatology, 1986.

J. Janne in 1985 demonstrated that the toxic anti-cancer drug MGBG was stopped from damaging cancer cells in experimental animals by carnitine. However, it did protect the animals from a toxic death by MGBG.

****

BIOFLAVONOIDS

Bioflavonoids are a complex of substances such as hesperidin and rutin. The primary source is in the white pulp of citrus fruits and is also found in apricots, plums, grapes, blackberries, etc. In medicine it has been recognized for many decades that bioflavonoids are responsible for maintaining the integrity of small blood vessels. When an individual develops black and blue marks easily, the use of Bioflavonoids quickly remedies the problem. Toxic copper is also removed from the body by bioflavonoids.

Quercetin, which is another bioflavonoid, was shown by M. Yoshida et al to inhibit the growth of human cancer cells.

A synthetic derivative, **flavone acetic acid** (FAA) was shown by D.J. Kern et al., in the British journal Cancer in 1989 to have a boosting effect on the immune system.

It was shown by R.L. Hornung et al. that (FAA) possessed natural killer cell activity in mice (not in people) .

MC Bibby et al., showed that this synthetic substance had an immunological effect. However, as a drug it was felt it wouldn't be useful against cancer. When will they ever learn? Every time scientists think that they can improve on nature's compounds with a synthetic, they are doomed to fail!

Flavone   acetic acid, when used in combination with interleukin-2, did have a positive effect on **kidney cancer** in mice, as well as, in people. I occasionally wonder what would be the effect on the use of natural bioflavonoids in combination with many of the substances discussed in this book, as compared to all of these artificial, profit making compounds and their toxic effects. And then I remember the experience of many years with patients and the wondering stops. Success for nature means doom for business! Take natural bioflavonoids!

****

VITAMIN C

Vitamin C has received more attention than any other vitamin as a preventive and treatment for cancer. Due mainly to the research and writings of Dr Linus Pauling, the only scientist to win two Nobel Prizes in Science, millions throughout the world are taking large doses for cancer and many other diseases. The Mayo clinic did a "test" of Dr. Pauling's claims that lasted only ten weeks and then publicly denounced him. This type of fraudulent counter-attack is typical of the tactics used against many reputable scientists over the centuries. Millions died needlessly until the truth finally emerged. Unfortunately, many excellent treatments have been buried because of the threats of the scientific establishment and governments against the "free" press. Literally thousands of scientific papers, have been written backing up all that Dr. Pauling has presented.

Most fruits, particularly citrus, contain large amounts of vitamin C. Many vegetables such as broccoli, tomatos, peppers are also excellent sources. Remember, however, taking antacids prevents absorption and smoking depletes vitamin C in the body. Dr. E. Schneider (Deutsch Med. Wchnschr. '54) noted significant improvement, prolongation of life and reduction of tumor size in patients placed on just 1,000 mgm of vitamin C and massive doses of vitamin A, 300,000 units intravenously for 281 doses. There were no untoward effects. Much evidence exists that vitamin E and A, in fact, adding a full complement of vitamins to vitamin C, has a beneficial effect. To rely on vitamin C alone would be erroneous.

W. J. McCormick in his article, "Cancer: A Preventable Disease, Secondary to Nutritional Deficiency?" (Clinical Physiology 1963), argues the point strongly. Four years earlier he had written in the Archives of Pediatrics that taking vitamin C was "an ounce of prevention, worth a pound of cure".

O. Bodansky and his group confirmed that deficiency of vitamin C existed in cancer cases.

Dr. Jorgen U. Schnegel, Chairman of Tulane University's Department of Urology, advocated 1,500 mg of vitamin C daily to prevent recurrences of bladder cancer. I had bladder cancer 22 years ago, guess what I have been doing? I take 3,000 mg and have taken as much as 18,000 mg daily of Dr. Pauling's famous recommendation for active cancer.

The world renowned, Dr. Max Gerson, strongly advocated the intake of vegetables rich in vitamin C.

I would be amiss if I did not mention that papers have been written in journals, almost too numerous to count, on the benefits of vitamin C in heart disease, hypertension, colds, polio, hepatitis and many other conditions (Frederick R. Klenner, M.D., in the Journal of Applied Nutrition, Winter Issue, 1971, VITAMIN C).

It is interesting that the recommended daily allowance (RDA) by the USA Government for vitamin C is 60 mg. They strangely caution pregnant and lactating women to limit their intake to 100 mg. Doctors recommend 100 to 200 mg a day in infections, after surgery, accidents and in smokers. In scurvy, the only vitamin C deficiency disease recognized by medicine, the Merck Manual recommends 1000 mg.

E. Kolb in Z. Gesamte Inn Med. 1984, noted a decrease in the ability of white blood cells to destroy bacteria.

Linus Pauling in an article submitted to the Proceedings of the National Academy of Sciences of the USA in 1976 recommended 10 to over 20 grams of vitamin C (1 gram = 1,000 mg), for all adults in order to inhibit the growth of cancer, improve general well-being and extend life. Pauling points out that humans are one of the few animal species that does not produce its own supply of vitamin C. Compared to other animals he states that the amount he recommends is normal. The clinical experiments carried out by Pauling and Cameron in Scotland in 1978 and 1979 on over a thousand patients revealed that survival time in cancer could be increased by more than 400 % over those who did not receive vitamin C.

In a study of lung cancer patients the beneficial effects included an increase in survival time of 3 to 4 months along with "symptomatic relief and improved sense of well-being". Although two Mayo Clinic studies refuted Pauling's claims (E. Creagan et al., New England Journal of Medicine, 1979 and C. Moertel et al. New England Journal of Medicine, 1985), there is strong evidence of invalid techniques used and other serious deficiencies in the Mayo Clinic studies. No patients died while receiving the vitamin C, but only after abrupt termination. Pauling and C. Herman argued this position in the Proceedings of the National Academy of Sciences in 1989. New Scientist, produced an article in which it was believed that some of the control subjects in the Mayo experiment were taking vitamin C on their own. There were also questionable practices by the Mayo Clinic. They placed participants in the study on 5-FU, a drug that is virtually useless in advanced cancers of this type, after they had been discontinued from taking the vitamin C. The failure of the Mayo Clinic to follow a specific protocol and then claim failure is tantamount to blatant fraud.

Since that time the evidence is accumulating that vitamin C as well as vitamin E and other anti-oxidants are unquestionably beneficial against cancer. J.H. Weisburger and C.L. Horn, in the Scandinavian Journal of Gastroenterology, 1984 indicate that the risk of **gastric cancer** can be decreased by vitamin C and these other supplements. They are particularly useful against foods which contain nitrites.

In laboratory mice with **Leukemia** survival time was increased by 70 % using vitamin C and B12 (H.F. Pierson, et al., Cancer Research, 1985).

A carcinogenic chemical found in pickled vegetables in China, RRME, was inhibited by large doses of vitamin C and retinamide (vitamin A derivative) from its damaging affects. This study was published in China in 1986.

The respected journal, Nature, in 1980 published an article showing that vitamin C killed **malignant melanoma** cells in the laboratory.

In 1990 M. Osmak achieved similar results with a vitamin C derivative.

Cancer Research in 1983 had an article by H.F. Pierson and G.G. Meadows which showed that the life-span of mice with **melanoma** could be significantly extended by the use of vitamin C, two amino acids (phenylalanine and tyrosine) and levodopa, a Parkinsonism drug.

Abraham Hoffer, MD, a famous Canadian scientist, who also did work with Linus Pauling, showed that survival of cancer patients could live as much as 16 times longer if they followed a complete nutritional program that included 10 g of vitamin C and beta-carotene daily. Their study was published in the Journal of Orthomolecular Medicine, 1990. In **cancer of the ovary, tubes and breast** the results were extremely impressive.

The National Cancer Institute held a symposium on ascorbic acids in 1990. Scientists from around the world were represented. Dr. Balz Frei of the University of California, Berkeley, presented a paper that showed that cancer chemical reactions could not take place in the presence of vitamin C.

E. Niki of Tokyo has produced a series of papers published between 1984 and 1987 that stressed the role of anti-oxidants, especially vitamin E and C in the control of harmful free radicals.

S. Harakeh in 1990 published in the proceedings of the National Academy of Sciences evidence that vitamin C interferred with the production of protein in infected cells by viruses (including HIV, the so-called Aids virus).

M.E. Poydock in a series of papers wrote of the affect of vitamin C and B12 on mitotic activity in mice with ascites tumors (Experimental Cell Biology, 1979, 1982, 1985).

Vitamin C was also shown to inhibit the incidence of kidney tumor which were brought on by the use of female sex hormones by Dr. Joachim Liehr of the University of Texas.

The list of studies is almost endless. As an indication of just a fraction of what has been studied with reference to vitamin C, I will list the investigator and subject of the study in very brief form;

Dr. Gary Meadows, Washington State University, vitamin C inhibits cancer growth in mice and augments affect of chemotherapy.

Dr. Jacob, San Francisco, low levels of blood vitamin C associated with increased levels of mutagenic substances related to colorectal cancer in stools.

Dr. Okunieff, radiation therapy for animals with cancer reduced by 50 %.

Dr. Gladys Block, National Cancer Institute, high level of blood vitamin C reduced cancer risk by 50 %.

Hiroshi Kan Shimpo, Fujiti Health University, vitamin C blocks heart muscle damage caused by chemotherapeutic and immunotherapeutic agents (adriamycin and interleukin-2).

Peter Wiernick, Montefiore Medical Center, New York, interleukin-2 causes massive decrease in vitamin C blood levels.

R. V. Birk, et al., Eksp. Onkol. 1988, demonstrated an adverse effect from vitamin C when the carcinogen, N-nitrosodiethylamine, was given to rats. (This is a classical example of combining two chemicals and using a dangerous drug in combination to try to discredit the role of vitamin C as a cancer preventive and treatment). A study done with **three** patients in which they developed potentially harmful symptoms while taking high doses of vitamin C for Hodgkin's disease and lung cancer, prompted caution that high levels of vitamin C be reached gradually.

S. Fukushima, Nagoya City University Medical School demonstrated that 5 times the vitamin C dose recommended by Pauling could accelerate the effects of bladder cancer. He originally used the sodium form of vitamin C but then later reported that the same extremely high dose of **ordinary ascorbic acid did not have an adverse effect on bladder cancer.**

S.M. Cohen, Cancer Research 1991, demonstrated that ascorbic acid did not promote tumors but that the sodium and other type of salts of many compounds did.

In spite of all the claims that vitamin C promotes kidney stones, D. du Bruyn demonstrated that very high doses of ascorbic acid over a 20 months period did not cause any deposition of crystals (stones) in 16 baboons.

This finding was confirmed by P.P. Singh, Journal of Urology, 1988 in their study with rats.

There are with vitamin C, as well as with purified drinking water a possibility of toxic reactions and even death. The extremes, however, to which one must go is rarely if ever, reached, even under the most unusual circumstances.

****

VITAMIN D

Vitamin D requires exposure to sunlight in order to be manufactured by the body. The Garland brothers proposed that sunlight is actually protective against the dreaded skin cancer, **malignant melanoma.** This is of course contrary to what is commonly thought about cancers of the skin and sunlight. Their premise was based on the fact the **melanomas occurred mostly in sailors who worked indoors and far less in those who worked outdoors.** Laboratory work had already shown that vitamin D suppressed melanoma growth. Their findings are represented in the Archives of Environmental Health, 1990.

A similar relationship seems to exist with **breast cancer** also. They presented an hypothesis involving exposure to solar radiation and geographic relationships in Preventive Medicine 1990. They concluded that the risk of fatal breast cancer in major cities was "inversely proportional to intensity of local sunlight".

The relationship of vitamin D, its dependency on sunlight for its formation and the occurrence of breast cancer was confirmed by E. D. Gorham in the Soviet Union and was published in the International Journal of Epidemiology in 1990.

Gorham also studied the "Acid Haze", which is caused by the high levels of sulfur dioxide in smog. Sulfur dioxide absorbs ultraviolet light and therefore, inhibits production of vitamin D in the skin. The incidence of death from breast and colon cancer was increased in 20 Canadian cities which suffered from air pollution. His finding were published in the Canadian Journal of Public Health in 1989.

E. A. Jacobson, in Cancer Research 1989, in a study on 40 rats placed on a high fat diet, found that lowered amounts of vitamin D and calcium promoted the development of breast cancer.

There is some evidence that receptors for vitamin D on cancer cell surfaces may actually inhibit their growth (K.W.

Colston, Lancet 1989).

R. Frampton in 1983 in Cancer Research showed that vitamin D in high doses actually changed cancer cells and suppressed their growth. The vitamin D hormone (D3) injected into mice with Leukemia, increased their survival time. It should be remembered that both vitamin D and the hormone D3 can be highly toxic and this should be seriously considered before ingesting more than 50.000 units a day.

I. N. Sergeev, in the Journal of Nutrition, indicated that **vitamin D must be accompanied by vitamin C** if it is to be truly beneficial. This has been confirmed by the Academy of Medical Scientists in Moscow.

John Ott, the well known researcher in light, maintains that the exposure to whole spectrum solar radiation is necessary for stimulation of the hypothalamus gland and for maintaining mental and physical health. He has produced full spectrum indoor artificial light to supplement the lack found in many remote parts of the world.

****

VITAMIN D AND CALCIUM

The incidence of colorectal cancer is reduced by two thirds in individuals who have a high vitamin D and calcium content in their diet. Studies done by doctors Frank and Cedric Garland at the University of San Diego School of Medicine over a nineteen year period showed that in men who ate **a diet rich in calcium and vitamin D had an incidence of colorectal cancer of 14.3 per 1000 as compared to 38.9 per 1000 in individuals who ingested low levels of these two nutrients.** This study was performed on 2000 men at the naval health research center in San Diego.

Because vitamin D levels are to a great degree determined by the exposure to sunshine studies have indicated a lower level of colorectal cancer in Western and Southern states.

****

VITAMIN E

Vitamin E has long been thought to be the anti-sterility vitamin. This is because it was initially found that a deficiency of Vitamin E caused sterility in mice. In recent decades, research has produced evidence that Vitamin E is not only beneficial for the heart and circulatory system, but it is a **protective against cancer**. Studies done on **mammary** dysplasia, a precursor to malignant breast disease in women, revealed that it affected the balance of estradiol, estriol and progesterone in the blood. These hormones are usually low in women who have mammary dysplasia.

Studies performed at the North Charles General Hospital in Baltimore, and published by R.S. London in Cancer Research, 1981, indicated that Vitamin E therapy could reduce risk of **breast cancers**. The same scientists reported in the Journal of the American College of Nutrition, 1983 and 1984 and the Journal of Reproductive Medicine in 1987, that Vitamin E was effective in reducing premenstrual symptoms (PMS).

K.N. Prasad and P.J. Edwards wrote in Cancer Research, 1982, that one of the forms of Vitamin E (tocopherol acid succinate) inhibited the growth of **melanoma cells** and suggested its possibility as a therapeutic agent for tumors.

I. D. Cappel, et al, in Anti-cancer Research, 1983, demonstrated that Vitamin E could reduce the toxicity of chemotherapy.

I. Szczepanska, et al, performed laboratory studies on human blood in test tubes and found that the addition of Vitamin E protected the cells from toxicity, from six out of the seven chemotherapeutic agents.

Chemotherapy and total body irradiation are given as conditioning therapy for individuals receiving bone marrow transplants (BMT). These patients were found to have low levels of Beta-Carotene and Vitamin E. M.R. Clements, et al, in a 1989 Free Radical Research Communication, recommended the use of these two antioxidants to all patients receiving BMT conditioning therapy.

B. LeGardeur, et al., and J. Stam, in articles published in Nutrition and Cancer, 1990, and Lung, 1990, respectively, reported that Vitamin E levels in the blood were low in patients with **lung cancer.**

D.G. Bespalov, et al., found that Vitamin E reduced the incidence of **digestive tract tumors** in 90% of the rats that had been given a strong carcinogen. Vitamin E and Selenium were found to work more effectively together in their anti-cancer activity.

C. Ip, in a letter to Cancer in 1985, stated that he felt Vitamin E was even more important than Selenium.

P. Knekt, et al., reported low levels of Vitamin E and Beta-Carotene in patients with **Melanoma.** In two articles published in the International Journal Epidemiology in 1988 and 1989, Knekt reported that low levels of Vitamin E in women had a 150% greater chance of developing cancer when compared with women with high levels of Vitamin E. A similar study done in over 20,000 men in Finland, revealed a similar effect. These studies lead Knekt and his group to conclude that Vitamin E protects against cancer. Further studies by Knekt on **cancers of the gastrointestinal tract**, revealed a relationship between low levels of Selenium and Vitamin E and the incidence of cancer in this area.

J. H. Williams, a South African Veterinarian, reported that the essential fatty acids (EFA) and gamma linolenic acid (GLA) were useful in the treatment of lymphoma in dogs. They also used Vitamin E in conjunction with their treatment.

Nitrosamines, which are formed by the body by the ingestion of nitrates, are inhibited in their formation by Vitamin E and Vitamin C. (D. Lathia and A. Blum, International Journal of Vitamin and Nutritional Research, 1989).

Research performed at the University of Colorado showed that vitamin E inhibits the growth of prostate cancer cells in the laboratory. The immune stimulating affect of vitamin E and it's neutralizing affect on free radicals protect the integrity of DNA.

****

VITAMIN K

The role of Vitamin K in the body, mainly centers around liver function and the ability of the blood to form a clot. Evidence is mounting, however, that Vitamin K is an

anti-cancer agent. (A. Mohsen, et al., Pharmazie. 1978; K.N. Prasad, et al. Life Sciences, 1981 and R.T. Chlebowski, et al., Cancer Treatment Review, 1985).

Chlebowski demonstrated that Vitamin K3 completely inhibited a certain form of mouse leukemia. When he combined Vitamin K and Warfarin, a rat poison to "thin the blood", he was able to inhibit the formation of cancers of the **liver, kidney, stomach, colon, ovary, breast, bladder, lung and melanoma.**

W. C. Su, et al., confirmed that K3 was effective in the treatment of **liver cancer** in experiments performed in Taiwan in 1991. Anti-cancer drugs can be enhanced in their activity by the addition of Vitamin K3.

L.M. Nutter, in Biochemical Pharmacology, 1991, stated that Vitamin K3 had "a broad spectrum of anti-cancer activity".

H. Osswald, et al., in Toxicology, 1987, also reported that this vitamin, when used in conjunction with toxic anti-cancer drugs, increased the life-span of mice with cancer.

When combined with Vitamin C, a single injection of anti-cancer drugs was markedly potentiated and was noted by H.S. Taper in the International Journal of Cancer, 1987.

****

MINERALS

CALCIUM

Just mention of the word, Calcium, brings images of bones and teeth to everyone. However, Calcium plays a role in the metabolism of the parathyroid gland, nerves, muscles and the clotting mechanism of blood. Calcium also plays an integral role in the metabolism of Vitamin D. It rarely works alone, however, and is found involved with the activities of Vitamins A, C, D, E, and other minerals (magnesium and phosphorus).

It is generally recognized that most of us suffer from a calcium deficiency in our diets. The incidence of osteoporosis is women, is alarmingly high and results from the slow process of calcium loss. There is some evidence that high blood pressure and elevated cholesterol levels are also related to calcium metabolism. D. A. McCarron, et al., in Medical Hypotheses, 1990, discussed the many difficulties in dealing with this calcium deficiency.

C.F. Garland, et al., in the American Journal of Clinical Nutrition, 1991, showed the relationship between low calcium and **colon cancer**. Supplementation of the diet with Vitamin D and calcium resulted in major reductions in cancer of the **rectum and colon**.

The role of **low fat, increased fiber** and **calcium** lowered the risk of these cancers (J.H. Weisburger and C.L. Horne, Scandinavian Journal of Gastroenterology Supplement, 1984).

In articles in the New England Journal of Medicine, 1985 and Cancer Research, 1989, M. Lipkin indicated that calcium supplementation reduced the proliferation of abnormal cells in individuals at high risk for **colon cancer**.

M. Buset, et al., in Cancer Research, 1986, confirmed Lipkin's findings. In articles in Cancer Research, 1986 and again in 1990, Buset demonstrated that calcium could block the **toxicity of certain fats**, known to be damaging and carcinogenic to the **colon**.

Studies in experimental rats showed that a high fat, low Vitamin D, low calcium diet, doubled the incidence of **breast cancer** (E.A. Jacobson, et al., Cancer Research, 1989).

****

CESIUM

The mineral, Cesium, is in an alkaline metal, present all over the earth but in tiny amounts. Radioactive Cesium seeds have been implanted in cancer patients, as a form of therapy. It is claimed to protect against radiation toxicity and, therefore, is used in conjunction with the radioactive implants. (E. Braverman, et al., Medical Hypotheses, 1988).

Ordinary Cesium has also been used as a treatment for cancer. This treatment is based upon elevating the pH into the alkaline range (above 7 which is neutral). the therapeutic approach advocated is referred to as the "high pH" therapy (alkaline) which endangers the life of the cancer cell, but is tolerated by normal cells. Cancer cells have an acidic pH (below 7) and it is felt that Cesium would neutralize the toxicity of the cancer cell (H.E. Sartori, Pharmacological Biochemical Behavior, 1984). In this article, Sartori cites the production of large amounts of mucous by the cancer cell which protects it from attack. He relies on the pharmacologic effect of many foods and recommends the macrobiotic approach, not too different from the more tolerable approach offered in this book. It was the low incidence of cancer in certain regions that prompted the use of alkali metals, i.e. cesium and rubidium. The therapeutic program consists of:

Antioxidants	**Cesium**	**Diet**
Essential FattyAcids	**Liver Oils**	**Minerals**
Oxygenation	**Potassium**	**Rubidium**
Sodium	**Vitamins**	

Cesium was demonstrated to reduce the growth of **Sarcomas** in mice. It was felt that Cesium replaced the potassium in cancer cells and, thus, interfered with their metabolism (A. El Domeira, et al., Journal of Surgical Oncology, 1981).

Studies done by F.S. Massiha indicated that there was a delicate balance that had to be maintained between the minerals, potassium and cesium in order for an anti-cancer effect to occur. When cesium and potassium are given together, the impact on **liver cancer** cells in rats was greater.

When combined with zinc gluconate in Vitamin A, **colon cancer** in mice was repressed (M.J. Tufte, et al., Pharmacological Biochemical Behavior, 1984).

Uptake of cesium is enhanced by zinc, selenium and Vitamins C and A.

Rubidium fed to mice along with cesium increased the destruction of tumor mass markedly and also markedly decreased the amount of pain the a study done on humans.

Studies on mice, in which tumors had been transplanted into the abdomen, Cesium Chloride has been tested on patients with terminal cancer. It was used along with other minerals, vitamin, chelating agents. The types of cancer on which it was used covered a wide spectrum and included **cancers of the gall**

bladder, liver, pancreas, lung, breast, prostate, sarcoma and lymphoma. H.E. Sartori reported this remarkable study in Pharmacological Biochemical Behavior in 1984. Although one quarter of the terminal patients died within the first two weeks, pain was markedly diminished (in many cases completely) and autopsies revealed that the cancer was eliminated in most of the cases.

C. Pinski and R. Bose, in the same journal, pointed out that if supplements and an adequate diet were used in conjunction with Cesium, toxicity was reduced considerably.

F. Messiha, at the same time, performed an experiment on rats with liver cancer which showed that alcohol administered with the Cesium reduced the toxicity by fifty percent.

****

GERMANIUM

Since the mid-seventies, when Japanese scientists synthesized an organic compound of Germanium, called Ge-132, studies have appeared indicating that Germanium has an **immune enhancing and anticancer effect**. Germanium is found in most foods and in water in minute amounts. In the late 1980's, its popularity grew in the United States and Europe. The well known medical journal, Lancet, published an anonymous article warning of its dangers, even though it gave no solid evidence.

Much of the research on Germanium has taken place in Japan. J. Satoh and T. Iwaguchi published a study on **liver cancer** in rats. They stated that Ge-132 had no cytotoxicity and that it did not destroy cancer cells directly. They credited activation of the immune system and reported "remarkable life prolongation". They were adamant in their opinion on its anti-tumor activity.

Their findings were confirmed in the United States by investigators, Y. Mizushima, et al., who reported in the International Archives of Allergy and Applied Immunology , 1980, that Ge-132 repaired immune responses and had a beneficial effect on the circulatory system.

Other studies on mice with **lung cancer**, who were administered Ge-132 with the anti-cancer agent 5-FU, showed that tumor growth was inhibited and metastatic spread was decreased. Survival time was increased and body weight of the mice was maintained.

H. Kobayashi and T. Munakata studied Ge-132, bleomycin and interferon in combinations that revealed a potentiating effect.

F. Suzuki, at the University of Texas, reported in The International Journal of Immunotherapy, 1986, confirmation of Ge-132 as an immuno-potentiating agent.

An anti-metastatic effect was confirmed by N. Kumano, et al., and published in the Journal of Experimental Medicine in 1985. It appears that the dose of Ge-132 determines its effect on metastases, and in **large doses could actually increase the number of metastases.**

N. Kumano, et al., in The Journal of Experimental Medicine, 1985, demonstrated that a **single dose of Germanium slowed the appearance of a metastatic tumor.**

J. J. Jang and his group in Carcinogenesis 1991, reported a positive effect on **lung and thyroid** cancers and, when Ge-132 was combined with garlic and an extract from cabbage called indoles, it was effective in the treatment of **liver cancer** in rats.

L. Pronai demonstrated that Ge-132 had a stabilizing effect on cell membranes and on white blood cell activity.

Kidney damage has been reported in studies by A. Schauss, T. Nakano and T. Matsusaka in various journals.

However, T. Sanai and S. Okuda reporting in the Journal, Kidney International, 1991, and Current Therapeutic Research, 1987, showed that the damage to kidneys occurred with the use of germanium oxide and not Ge-132. Because of the fear of malpractice suites, alternative therapists have been extremely cautious in the use of germanium. Germanium dioxide sometimes contaminates Ge-132 during its manufacture and careful monitoring of kidney function should be carried out during its administration.

****

LITHIUM

Lithium is currently the standard psychiatric chemotherapy

for manic-depressive psychosis. It is potentially very toxic and must be continuously and carefully administered under the supervision of a physician. Dr. Hans Neiper, the famous German physician, has been using **lithium orotate (450 mg/day)** and finds this amount extremely safe in contrast to lithium carbonate, Aggressology 1973.

Lithium has also been used to counteract the decrease in white blood cells and infections that occur during cancer chemotherapy (G.H. Lyman, et al., New England Journal of Medicine, 1980).

P. B. Steinhertz in the Journal of Pediatrics and R. Pazdura in the journal, Blood, 1981, confirmed this effect on the white blood cells.

M.P. Spina of Italy, demonstrated that this sparing effect on white blood cells was long term.

S. Molnar demonstrated that lithium had the ability to stimulate the maturation of white blood cells in the bone marrow.

A. Ballin at the Tel Aviv University, published an article in the British Journal of Cancer in 1983, that indicated that the chemotherapeutic agents, bleomycen and vinblastine, in conjunction with lithium, was greatly enhanced in their ability to delay the appearance of tumors, kill tumor cells and extend survival time in mice with melanoma.

Tumor necrosis factor and lithium worked synergistically in activating white blood cell action against cancer cells.

F. Witz, of Paris, and G.H. Lyman, of Tampa, Florida, have both indicted lithium toxicity as a risk for sudden death, usually of heart problems, in cancer patients.

****

MAGNESIUM

Magnesium has gained significant notice since the famous international cardiologist, Dmitri Sodi-Pollares of Mexico, lectured and published on its incredible beneficial effect in most heart disease. Magnesium has since been advanced as part of a combination of supplements in the treatment of cancer.

In a study published in the Japanese Journal of Cancer

Research, rats which were exposed to a carcinogen that caused **breast cancer** in rats, were administered various combinations of **magnesium, selenium, vitamin C and vitamin A.** When given a common combination of all four, the reduction in the appearance of tumors was decreased by 88% and the number of tumors also declined (A. Ramesha, Japanese Journal of Cancer Research, 1990).

J.M. Blondell in Medical Hypotheses, 1980, proposed that magnesium produced its effect by maintaining the fidelity of genetic material and the membranes of cells thus guarding against the onset of cancerous changes.

****

MOLYBDENUM

Molybdenum is essential for the formation of enzymes which play a significant role in the oxidation of fats and the release of iron from the liver. The deficiency of molybdenum in the soil determines its level of availability in our food.

C. S. Yang in Cancer Research, 1980, believed that molybdenum deficiency was part of a complex of problems that lead to wide spread **esophageal cancer** in China. The addition of molybdenum and vitamin C to the diet decreased the incidence of this dreaded cancer.

Addition of minute amounts to drinking water significantly inhibits the development of **esophageal and stomach cancer** (X.M. Luo, Journal of the National Cancer Institute, 1983). Molybdenum added to drinking water, reduced by 50% the occurrence of **breast cancer** in rats, who were exposed to a carcinogen.

The study performed by H.J. Wei in 1987, also demonstrated that tungsten, an antagonist to molybdenum, promoted breast tumors.

M. P. Kopf in 1979, achieved 100% tumor inhibition for thirty days, in mice who had received a transplantation of tumor cells.

****

SELENIUM

Dr. Emmanuel Revici, the incredible octogenarian cancer therapist of New York, has used selenium for over fifty years. Because, like most other substances in life, too little or too much can be harmful, controversy exists over its use. Laboratory studies have shown that it is useful in providing protection against carcinogenic substances, viruses, ultra violet light and in its action against tumor cells.

J. Neve, in the journal of Clinical Endocrinological Metabolism, 1985, argued against its use. However, H. S. Ladas performed an extensive review of the literature and argued strongly in favor of selenium (Holistic Medicine, 1989).

Many theories exist as to the mechanisms by which selenium works as an effective therapy in cancer. These theories include DNA repair, protection of the genes, elimination of free radicals, inhibition of tumor growth, activation of natural killer cells (H.T. Petrie, University of Nebraska Medical Centre, 1988, Doctorate dissertation).

Elevated levels of selenium in the diet, correlate with a lower incidence of **cancers of the breast, lung, pancreas, ovary, rectum, prostate, bladder and skin** (G. Schrauzer, Bio-organic Chemistry, 1975 and 1977).

Low selenium levels in the blood correlated with the occurrence of **stomach and lung cancer** in men and a relationship was shown with breast cancer in women (P. Knekt, Journal of the National Cancer Institute, 1990 and H. Ksrnjavi, in Breast Cancer Research and Treatment, 1990).

The Chinese Academy of Medical Scientists found that selenium was a safe and effective food supplement and was useful for protection against carcinogenic substances and radiation from ultra violet light (S. Yu, Biological Trace Research , 1990,).

Selenium relies upon high levels of vitamin E to be effective (C. Ip, Cancer Lett. 1985). Emmanuel Revici advocates the use of 10,000 micrograms, as compared to the 150 micrograms of selenium recommended by the National Academy of Sciences. Revici's superb knowledge with reference to the balance of positive and negative biochemical forces, successfully and without danger, administers this very large dose of selenium along with fatty acids in organic substances. Revici bases his work, first on the determination of the "anabolic" or "catabolic" state of the patient and when the urine is alkaline (pH is above 7.0).

Revici's work involving several **organic selenium** compounds, have been confirmed by H. S. Ladas and K. Schwartz. Revici has written a medical text, Research in Physiopathology as Basis of Guided Chemotherapy, with Special Application to Cancer, Nostrand & Company, 1961.

It must be remembered that selenium, like any other substance, can be toxic when used excessively. The symptoms are easily recognized and include metallic taste, rashes, discolored teeth, hair loss, nervousness, depression, pallor and a heavy odor of garlic. Although many attempts have been made to discredit and discourage the use of selenium, they have been discounted by the World Health Organization and relate mainly to the inorganic form.

Laboratory studies appear to indicate that **cancer rates can be reduced by up to 70 percent by simply adding selenium, which is found in the soil, to our diet.** Our soil has become so depleted of this vital substance that we must now take it in supplemental form. **The National Cancer Institute believes that this ingredient is so vital that it should be included in the Recommended Daily Allowance (200 micrograms).** Vitamin E, increases the anticancer effect of selenium (Ip C., Cancer Letter. 1985)

The study published by J.H. Weisberger and C.L. Horn in the Scandinavian Journal of Gastroenterology indicate that selenium plus calcium and other micro-nutrients found in green and yellow vegetables, could lower the risk of **gastro-intestinal cancers.**

Selenium also enhances the absorption of potassium, rubidium and cesium by cancer cells thus facilitating therapy. It should be included in mineral supplementation.

The use of selenium in rats reduced the incidence of **breast cancer** 50%. When combined with magnesium, vitamin C and vitamin A the incidence was reduced 88% (A. Ramesha, Japanese Journal of Cancer Research, 1990)

****

TELLURIUM

Tellurium, although a very toxic element, has proved to be effective against cancer and in stimulating the production of interleukin-2. This was successfully accomplished when a synthetic organic tellurium compound was developed in the late 1980's. This compound, AS 101, has been found to increase white blood cells, anti-cancer cytokines, colony stimulating factor (CFS), tumor necrosis factor (TNF) and has been sited for its immuno-regulatory function.

B. Sredni in Nature, 1987, and again in Immunology, 1990, wrote of many of the potential therapeutic applications. D. J. Alcocer and M. Blank wrote of the beneficial role of AS 101 in the treatment of systemic lupus erythematosus.

Many toxic effects have been noted, but investigator A. Nyska, believes that a selenium-vitamin E deficiency may be responsible for some of them. Warning! More is not better.

****

ZINC

Zinc is a truly remarkable mineral and has gained notoriety from books written about its use in sore throats and in prostatic enlargement and infection.

J. P. Larue, in the Journal of Urology, 1985, demonstrated that the level of zinc in the prostate gland was very high.

M.P. Waalkes and his group studied the action of zinc against the carcinogenic mineral Cadmium. Zinc markedly reduced tumor incidence caused by cadmium and the larger the amount of zinc used, the less the incidence of **testicular cancer** (Cancer Research 1989).

Several studies have investigated the low level of zinc in **prostate cancer** (A. Leake, Acta Endocrinol, Copenhagen, 1984).

Although zinc may play an important role in the treatment of prostate cancer, the occurrence of prostate cancer appears to be more dependent on a high intake of dietary fat (J. Ogunlewe, Cancer, 1989; K. E. Tvedt, Prostate, 1989; M.Y. Heshmat, Prostate 1985; and D.W. West, C.C.C. 1991).

Chapter 8

When The People Fight Back - Victory!

714-X (NITROAMINOCAMPHOR)

Gaston Naessens, a renowned biologist, is the developer of Nitramoniocamphor (714-X). A political battle erupted in Canada over its use as a treatment for cancer. Dr. Naessens won his battle against the medical establishment because his treatment had successfully defeated cancer in the relatives of some of the most prominent political figures in Canada. It is, of course, still outlawed in the United States. Dr. Naessen's view of cancer and its treatment is one that rejects the establishments' illogical position that it is a cellular disease isolated from general biologic disorders. He firmly believes, as all holistic or advanced scientists, that the evolution of cancer is linked to, and solely dependent on the organism in which it grows. He rejects the use of radiation, surgery and chemotherapy because they are directed at the result of the problem rather than the cause. Moreover, they usually mutilate the organism, destroy normal tissue and suppress the body's ability to attack, contain and reverse the processes responsible for the cancer.

He correctly reasons that we are all, for the most part, exposed to the numerous causes of cancer around us. Recognizing that this is indeed true, and in addition that many of us do not develop the disease, then is it not probable that there exists in those persons a resistance to cancer? Experiments have revealed that individuals stricken with cancer readily accepted tumor grafts from other individuals, whereas "normal" individuals did not. This remarkable event was directly opposite to the usual graft rejection one would have expected. The obvious explanation was that the cancer patients had lost the natural defense mechanisms that would have normally rejected the grafts. The same patients, however, did reject grafts of normal tissue. This indicated that the defenses dealing with cancerous tissue were different from those dealing with normal tissue. Other experiments have further shown that "normal" volunteers rejected grafts of cancerous tissue. There are obviously biochemical codes or sensors which, when destroyed or altered, can no longer signal a response by the immune system to attack the invader. They, in fact, adopt the identity of the foe (the cancer tissue) and will then act toward normal tissue as the enemy.

It is also known that the process of fermentation, which involves enzymes, causes the cell to revert to a more primitive state. This prevents differentiation and the cell reproduction falls into disarray and more rapid growth. The temperature, pH and pressure in the environment surrounding the cell, play an important role in cell growth. These aspects of the cell environment have been largely ignored. The experimentally produced variations of the chemistry of the environmental fluids have failed to reproduce the symptoms of acute and chronic diseases. Attention was focused on the tumors themselves and remedial efforts have therefore never dealt with the cause, only the results.

****

LOOKING FOR A SOLUTION

In his quest for an answer, Naessens developed an advanced microscope capable of magnifying 30,000 times (standard microscopes are capable of only 1,800 times magnification). This enabled him to observe carefully, an amazing phenomenon which has been written about extensively for over a century i.e. polymorphism (the ability to change form). There exists over one thousand scientific papers dealing with this occurrence involving frequently observed particles in the microscope field. Naessens has labeled them SOMATIDES. The Somatide is an extremely small elementary particle that moves by electromagnetic force. This is accomplished by negative repulsion, very much like what occurs when you turn a magnet around, and instead of attracting the paper clips, it pushes them away. The complete somatide cycle is illustrated in the figure that follows:

Figure 1: The Somatid Cycle

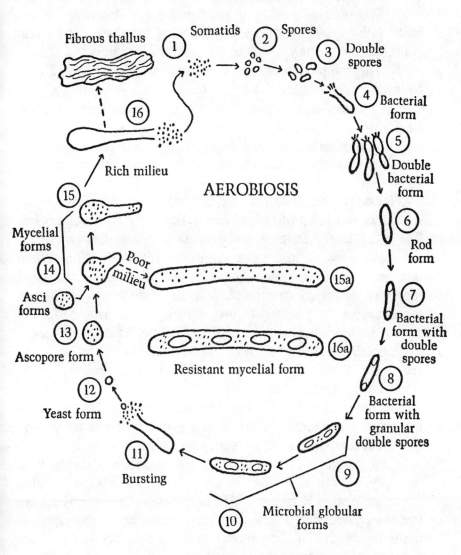

Naessens' discoveries give us a completely new and revolutionary approach to all disease processes, especially infection. His observations and research revealed:

A. In healthy individuals, only somatides, spores and double spores are observed (numbers 1 through 3 on diagram).

1. During this microcycle a proliferative hormone, **trephone,** which promotes multiplication of the cell, is detected. It is necessary for cellular division and therefore essential to life.

2. The production of trephone is controlled by inhibitors in the blood (mercury, copper, lead and other organic substances.

3. The process usually stops at this stage. However, if the balance is upset by **overproduction of trephone**, the cycle continues on through the other steps shown in figure 1.

B. The completion of the cycle involves passing through the following forms: bacterial > double bacteria > spore forming bacteria (yeast-like organisms) > fungal-like elements and finally to a pseudo-mycelial or branch-like structure, whose active cytoplasm, an internal cellular material, causes an eruption with the liberation of an enormous amount of new somatides.

Naessens then compares this pattern of activity to the reproductive cycles of the various types of cells in our bodies. The effect of the fermentation process in our bodies can revert the cellular cycles to a more primitive type of division. When this occurs the cell loses it individuality and function and therefore its ability to reproduce in its normal way. It cannot reproduce in the planned or programed genetic pattern. In this state it multiplies far more rapidly. Naessens refers to this stage as cancerization. If the "immune" system is intact, and can recognize these alien, "wild" and unlawful cells, it will immediately destroy them.

This development of foriegn cells apparently occurs daily, but the process is aborted before it gets started. This is the reason that precancerous lesions are easily corrected.

If the immune system is deficient, and aliens continue to multiply, a "critical mass" is achieved and a substance called Co-cancerogenic K factor (CKF) is released. CFK paralyzes the immune system and drains nitrogen from the body (the source is amino acids, the building blocks of protein) which is necessary for the proliferation of the cancer cell.

With this knowledge, Naessens was able to devise an approach based on neutralizing CKF. This led to the use of a camphor compound after testing many appropriate substances that were candidates for achieving this goal. Naessens chose camphor because it brings to cancer cells nitrogen without sacrificing normal cells and negating the need to produce CKF which paralyzes the immune system. The immune system is thus allowed to regain its ability to attack the cancer as a foriegn body. Camphor is classified as a terpene and is related in structure to quercetin, hesperidin, squalene and phytoene. It has been used internally as a stimulant and carminative. It has also been used as a preservative in pharmaceuticals. Although the action of camphor is not well understood, it falls into the phytochemical group which is known to protect against fungal and bacterial infections. Phytochemicals are good quenchers of oxygen-free radicals and are anti-carcinogenic, detoxifiers and enzyme regulators.

****

Chapter 9

The Universal Energy

ELECTROMAGNETIC THERAPIES

Fortuitously, in the early 1960's, I was exposed to a new treatment, called "trigger point" injections, which was started by Dr. Janet Travell. Dr. Travell, at that time, was the first woman to serve as a White House physician. She served President Kennedy and successfully helped him with his back pain. I had used this technique successfully for ten years, until Nixon went to China, at which time I realized that I had been doing Acupuncture, by injection without knowing it. This spurred my interest in expanding its use and in investigating other ancient techniques in medicine.

Acupuncture has been used in the Western World, primarily for the control of pain. It took many years for Western physicians to be even tolerant of its use and it was only accepted to a moderate degree when electrical stimulation of the points was utilized in hospitals and pain centres. Acupuncture, however, works well in other areas. Evidence has been collected that indicates it stimulates the immune responses in both infection, allergy and tumors. An equally ancient technique involves the use of points on the ear that, when stimulated, often give an even greater response. This technique, was originated in Ancient Egypt, and is referred to as Auriculotherapy. My thirty years of experience in this area as both a practitioner and teacher, has led me to the conclusion that these techniques are safe and effective adjuncts to therapy in cancer and other diseases, but must be used in conjunction with other natural therapies. Many excellent physicians of complementary medicine, homeopathy, naturopathy and chiropractics are adept in the use of these techniques, and are equipped to prescribe for a patient other natural therapies.

It is because acupuncture is an expression of electro-magnetic pathways of body energy flow and because the most common form in use today is accomplished with electrical stimulation, I have included it in this chapter.

****

ENVIRONMENTAL ELECTROMAGNETIC FACTORS

A number of years ago, I spent approximately six months in Phoenix, Arizona. During that time, I made several trips, a little over 100 miles north, to Sedona. Thirty-six years had passed since I interned at the Memorial Hospital in Phoenix, Arizona and I remembered the trip my wife and I made to beautiful Oak Creek Canyon where Sedona is located. Its enchanting beauty had stayed with me all those years, and so I was anxious to return. There was another reason. I had read several articles about geopathic zones and several scientists I knew, who were interested in electro-magnetic fields, had spoken of the powerful pathways of electrical fields which traverse the earth and have several meeting points all around the globe. Sedona is one of those places and it is believed by many to be capable of imparting a healing energy.

Geopathic Zones represent a relatively new area of study that gained impetus in the early 1920's, when a German oncologist, by the name of Sauerbruck, discussed the presence of low-frequency electromagnetic currents in the earth. Saurerbruck proposed that these currents could dramatically draw energy from the body thus resulting in an increase in the risk of developing cancer in individuals exposed to them. These concepts and theories were developed further by Dr. Ernst Hartmann of Eberbach, Germany in the early 1960's. Recent scientific studies have confirmed their observations. It is now known that very low electromagnetic frequencies of 5-25 Hz can cause cells to become cancerous. This frequency range is referred to as ELF (extremely low frequencies). It is believed they are caused by the flow of underground water, beneath the earth's surface. In recent years, Dr. Hans Nieper stated that more than 90% of all his cancer patients were exposed to ELF during their sleeping hours. Hundreds of papers have now appeared on this subject confirming that high tension wires, transformer stations and even electrical appliances, such as heating pans, electric blankets and clock radios can affect the body's normal function and the ability of the immune system to adequately defend against infection and genetic changes.

The amount of exposure to sun light, which is another form of electro-magnetic frequencies, likewise affects not only the immune system, but even our emotional state. Studies have shown that people who live in the far north, especially areas where the days become very short and the exposure to sunlight is even more limited by inclement weather, suffer from melancholia and depression to a much greater degree than the rest of the world's population. It has also been observed that immune defenses are reduced by as much as 30% during the end of August until the first frost. The rate of growth of malignancies increase dramatically during this period. These effects have been attributed to the passing of the solar system through dense electromagnetic fields. Many scientists believe that it is this phenomenon that accounts for the increase in upper respiratory infections rather than the weather.

The use of "excessive" heat in the home, above 18 degrees C. (64.5 degrees F.), has been demonstrated to cause suppression of the immune system. Saving energy takes on a double importance. I recall reading years ago that sudden changes of temperature over 15 degrees F. are capable of causing an allergic-like response of the body. It is further evidence that our environment, within and without, offers us the answers to staying healthy - and not the drugstore or the doctors office.

****

ELECTROMAGNETIC FIELD THERAPY

Electricity is only one of the aspects of electromagnetic

therapies. Electrical currents can produce a variety of effects and the conversion of electricity into magnetic fields, light spectrums and varying types of electrical currents are only the beginning of a very young science that has very old roots. B. Nordenstrom, of Sweden, is a modern physician pioneer, whose work clearly points to the fact that different forms of electromagnetic energy have varying effects on different types of tumors. At the risk of over-simplifying, if you can perceive that the essence of energy is vibration, then you can imagine that a particular vibration could selectively destroy a cancer cell while leaving normal cells unharmed. If you remember that all substances, in our Universe, have a positive or negative charge of varying degrees, you can further imagine that selective treatments can be based on counteracting or neutralizing that charge. It must be remembered, however, that many many of these techniques have already been shown to also cause serious damage. Our knowledge is sorely lacking because we have placed more faith in the curative powers of chemistry and ignored intensive investigation into the fields of energy. In the meanwhile humankind is suffering the carcinogenic effects of electricity, microwave, radio waves, ultra violet, x-rays and nuclear radiation.

****

ELECTRO-ACUPUNCTURE

NEUROPROBE

In this technique, the physician uses a source of direct current, as opposed to an alternating current, to stimulate the specific acupuncture points indicated. The major advantage is that the stimulation time is only 30-60 seconds, thus allowing the treatment of many points in a brief period. There are acupuncture points which are used to stimulate the immune system and to assist impaired function of the diseased organ. These points are not only located on the body, but on the ear as well (Auriculotherapy). The effectiveness of ear points has always impressed me more than body points in the thirty years I used it in my practice. An amazing phenomenon exist with

115

reference to the use of the ear diagnostically. It is possible to diagnose the existence of a "problem" area long before it appears clinically. This simple, but extremely accurate diagnostic technique can alert the physician to investigate early, a distinct advantage when it turns out to be a cancer.

T.E.N.S.

Transcutaneous Electrical Nerve Stimulation is commonly used in the world today in the treatment of neuromuscular disorders and pain syndromes. It is most effective when the therapist has knowledge of acupuncture. The usual practice of placing the electrode pads over the area of pain accounts for the poor results commonly obtained. The stimulation consists of alternating currents and takes approximately 30 minutes.

****

AUTHOR'S PREFERENCE

Injecting the acupuncture points with a non-toxic solution such as vitamin B12 and procaine has been in my experience superior to needling, heat, cold, pressure or electrical stimulation. The technique is almost painless, quick and has a stronger and longer-lasting effect. A few drops of the solution is injected less than a centimeter (1/4 inch) into the skin for most points. A 27 gauge needle, which is extremely fine is, used. In experienced hands the patient does not feel the stick!

****

PULSED ELECTROMAGNETIC ENERGY

(PEME)

After a 17 year battle with the FDA, the Diapulse Corporation, the original manufacturer of this remarkable machine, finally won in the courts. This technique has been used for decades successfully all over the world. In the United States no claims can be made other than in the area of pain, inflammation and healing of tissue, particularly bone fractures. I personally used PEME to stimulate the immune system as have so many physicians throughout the world. The Pharmaceutical industry and their brain-washed allies in establishment medicine, have stalled the progress to the future that this incredible energy promises. I have seen marvelous results in so many of the diseases in which establishment medicine does nothing but harm.

****

HYPERTHERMIA

Foolishly, patients and physicians alike, act quickly to eliminate the presence of fever in illness. We ignore the fact that fever is the obvious natural response of the body to combat unwanted intruders. This, not only applies to infection, but to a variety of irritants and **cancer** as well. The use of heat in medicine goes back to the Ancient Egyptians and frequently throughout history and in almost every culture, its use has been documented.

The National Cancer Institute has reported a positive response in **brain, head, neck, breast and skin cancers**, to heat therapy (National Cancer Institute, "Cancer Weekly", 29 May 1989). The benefits obtained from the different forms of electrical energy have been interpreted on the basis of the minimal amount of heat generated, rather than on the type of energy generated in wave lengths (the heat is often incidental).

M.M. Park in Lymphokine Research, 1990, reported that **microwaves** applied to the body, generated a small increase in body temperature, which induced immunological responses (a naive and incorrect assumption). The work of Robert Becker, who is probably the world's most renowned investigator in electro-magnetic medicine, has clearly outlined that various wavelengths cause different effects. The generation of heat, therefore, cannot be singled out from the source that generates it.

In experiments, in which the body heat is raised to 107 degrees, damage to cancer tissue, while essentially sparing normal tissue, has been demonstrated. Beneficial effects usually

117

occur best during the early stages of disease (H.I. Robbins and J.D. Cohen, Adv Exp Med. Biol.1990, H. S. Goldsmith and L. Stettiner, American Journal of Surgery, 1979, A. Dresnick, et al., Can J Surg.1982).

Hyperthermia, used in conjunction **with chemotherapy**, enhances the anti-tumor effect of chemotherapy (T. Tenaka, 1989, K. Hynen and B. A. Lulu, Investigative Radiology, 1990).

Articles have appeared in Lancet as early as 1979, in which scientists were attempting to raise the body temperature to dangerous levels, at the same time, hoping to spare normal tissue.

The work of A.R. Keen and R.W. Frelick demonstrated that natural body defenses are enhanced by fever (Del Med J. 1990).

Hyperthermia, generated by **radio frequencies**, was shown to be effective in metastatic cancer by R.E. Falk, et al., and reported in the Surg Gynecol Obstet, 1983.

Laser light energy, in both low and high intensity, and in many wavelengths, has been demonstrated to be effective against cancer and many other diseases (A.C. Steger, British Medical Journal, 1989).

High frequency sound waves (ultrasound) and magnets have also been used successfully in the treatment of brain tumors (H.I. Robbins, Semin Oncol. 1991; P.M. Harari, et al., Int J Radiat Oncol Biol Phys. 1991).

Radioactive substances have long been used in treating cancer and these too, are simply another form of electromagnetic energy. Combining heat with radiation, or chemotherapy, as well as all kinds of combinations of the various techniques mentioned, have been reported to increase the anti-cancer effect. Perhaps the chemotherapy can be discarded?

Scientific articles about electromagnetic therapies have appeared in the hundreds, in such varied publications as The American Journal of Clinical Oncology, The International Journal of Hyperthermia, Advanced Experimental Medical Biology, Medical Hypotheses, etc. The FDA, for decades has literally placed obstacles in the way of obtaining approval for medical devices that would obviate the use of drugs. The FDA is content to not only spend a fortune in obstructing advances in science, but, as usual, they coldly ignore substantial evidence, when presented by non-pharmaceutical interests. Meanwhile millions suffer and die. Make no mistake, the stringent requirements placed on the development of treatments for diseases in which we have failed to be effective therapeutically, does not protect the consumer. they merely give the pharmaceutical giants, who can afford the price tag, a monopoly at the exclusion of everyone else.

****

IONS

Far more than 5,000 scientific papers have been published on the effect of ions. Ions are particles that are electrically charged. They can be positive or negative and are the result of natural radiation from the sun, the earth, water, lightning and other atmospheric energy sources. It is known scientifically that negative ions freshen and revitalize the air. These ions are formed when an electron becomes attached to an oxygen molecule.

For several centuries, scientists have noted the effect of electricity in the atmosphere and its effect on vegetation (Father Gianbatista Beccaria of the University of Turin, late 18th Century). Bertholon, during the same period, wrote that electricity influenced the state of health and the course of a disease. At the end of the last century, Elster and Geitel of Germany and J.J. Thompson of England, discovered the presence of electrically charged particles in the air, which they called Ions. Seante Arrhenius, a Swedish student, eventually won the Nobel prize for a doctoral thesis which he had written years before and which had been ridiculed by science for proposing and theoretically proving the presence of ions.

The effect of cosmic rays, solar radiation, radioactive substances in soil, such as radon and Thoron, all produce ions directly or by striking the molecules of atmosphere and gas, causing them to lose or to gain electrons and, thus the molecule becomes positive or negative. Natural air sprays and waterfalls generate ion production. Both negative and positive ions can exist together in the air because they are separated by incredibly large numbers of molecules (ten quadrillion). Although the number of ions is extremely small compared with the number of

119

ordinary molecules in the air, modern science has proven the effect of extremely small currents and voltages on physiological and pathological process. Studies have shown many biological effects, including the deadly effect on micro-organisms, the stimulation of endocrine glands (adrenals, ovaries, testes, thyroid) and the production of enzymes, as well as the effect of ions on neuro-hormones in the brain with regard to circulation.

Professor Herbert Pole has done studies which prove that negative ions stimulate the growth of food plants and flowering plants. Experiments have demonstrated the difference between the ions and electrical fields. Recent discoveries have shown that there are various types of ions and that they have specific actions. The implications of this finding has almost unlimited possibilities. The level of many hormones, including the reproductive hormones, is markedly affected by the level of ionization in the air. Negative ions have been shown to have a beneficial effect on reproduction in laboratory animals.

Professor Felix Sulman at the Hadassah Medical School in Jerusalem, has demonstrated that negative ionized air can have a beneficial effect in the treatment of illnesses commonly caused by air that is positively ionized, such as the hot, dry winds (Sharab) which occur in Israel. The paving of streets, the air-conditioning and heating of our homes and the air trapped inside by well-insulated buildings, all inhibit or destroy negative ions.

Negative ion therapy has been used successfully in Russia by Drs. P.C. Bulatov and P.G. Portenov in Physical Therapy.

Dr. Ucha Udabe in Argentina, has used ion therapy effectively for anxiety syndromes.

Christian Bach of Denmark has used it environmentally with patients with asthma and hay fever.

Peter Fox of England has used it to treat migraine.

Dr. Deleanu of Romania has used this therapy for duodenal ulcers.

In the United States, Dr. I. Kornblueh, has found it beneficial in the treatment of patients with severe burns.

Ion generators are available for purchase. However, no claims can be made for them in the area of therapeutics because double-blind studies have not been done. It is unlikely that they will be done unless a source of funds for experiments of this nature, is made available. I, personally, use an ion generator in my room along with an ozone-producing ultra-violet light that is shielded because of the possible harmful effect of ultra-violet on the eyes.

The purpose of bringing the discussion of ions into cancer therapies is because the production of ions (particularly negative ions) brings about the following observed phenomena:

1. A small amount of ozone is produced thus cleansing the environment.

2. Dust, smoke and other particulate matter is precipitated out of the air.

3. Negative ions produce physical, mental and emotional uplift (Dr. Clarence Hansell, RCA Laboratories, 1932).

4. Improvement in general state of health, appetite and sleep. In three weeks there is a major increase in work capacity (Minkh, Russia).

5. Antibiotic effect and tissue repair enhancement and protection from pneumonia (Boyko, USSR; Deleanue,Romania; Balti, Israel).

6. Antifungal.

7. Analgesic effect (pain relief).

Considering all these effects, it is obvious that it is a major plus as an adjunct in prevention and treatment.

****

PHOTOTHERAPY

The use of light to treat disease is well documented in civilizations three and four thousand years ago. The Egyptians and the Greeks used sunlight and various colors in combination with plants. Red colored light has been the most frequently used light wavelength, as far back as Hippocrates. At the beginning of the 20th century, ultra violet light proved to be effective in the treatment of tuberculosis skin lesions. This discovery won a Nobel prize for M.R. Finsen in 1903.

The modern use of the color red was developed in 1937 in Germany with the use of hematoporphyrin (which is obtained from red blood cells) to sensitize cells to light. This treatment is still in use today and effectively destroys targeted cells. The ancient Egyptian combination of light and drugs has received considerable attention in the past decade and various combinations have proven effective.

The drug, 8-MOP, was originally studied by A.M. El Mofty in the 1940's. Almost fifty years later, Dr. R.L. Edelson discussed the very same drug in the treatment of a skin lymphoma (Scientific American 8, 1988).

D. Mew, et al., reporting in Cancer Research, 1985, demonstrated that photochemical agents, such as hematoporphyrin, were many times more powerful when used in conjunction with light.

This basic reaction provides a vehicle by which photosensitive dyes can be attached to drugs, antibodies, antigens and cells, so that the selective destruction of cancer cells can be obtained (H. Barr, et al., International Journal of Colorectal Disease, 1989; D.J. Castro, et al., Laryngoscope, 1991).

Hyperthermia has been combined with phototherapy and found to be effective against carcinoma (N. Matsumoto, et al., Arch Otolaryngol Head, Neck, Surg. 1990).

V. G. Schweitzer, in 1990, reported dramatic results in cancers of the head and neck. Effective combinations with drugs can be obtained while minimizing side effects (S.P. Zhao, et al., Ann Otol Rhiol Laryngol, 1990).

T. Okunka and his group demonstrated that phototherapy in combination with surgery, improved longevity in **lung cancer** patients.

Photopheresis involves removing blood from the body, treating it with light and returning it to the body. This process, which is extremely simple, and non-toxic, has long been known to be effective for infections when exposed to ultra violet light. Major universities, throughout the world, are currently studying its use, particularly in blood cancers. Doctors of advanced medicine have been exposed to information on the use of light in many diseases.

Because artificial light lacks important wavelengths, full spectrum light indoors is recommended, particularly for individuals who have cancer or evidence of immune suppression (J. Ott, Eye, Ear, Nose, Throat, Monograph 1974 and Ann Dent. 1968). (See Resourse Section)

****

TACHYON ENERGY - PULSORS

These are energy resonators which act as receivers and transmitters of specific frequencies of energy. A pulsor consists of millions of micro-crystals which receive, amplify and then re-transmit body energies with their own ordered pulse, hence the name pulsors. Some scientists believe that the earth contains an energy field of very high density. It is referred to as the Tachyon field and is a source of limitless energy. Tachyon crystals or beads are reported to harness this energy and transmit it to the body. This energy has been referred to as anti-entropic. Entropy is the word which refers to the tendency of any living system to follow an ever increasing path of disorder into death. An anti-entropic would therefore do just the opposite, i.e. create greater order and life. Just as a ordinary light bulb defuses light in all directions, a laser beam concentrates that light in an ordered form. Disease represents disorder, and health is proportional to a uniform state of ordered energy.

Therapeutic use of Tachyon beads is currently in its infant stages. Experiments have demonstrated an increase in performance of athletes, but as yet, to my knowledge, no controlled studies have been performed. There are individual case studies in which patients have exhibited and claimed all kinds of improvement, from reduction in pain, to improvement in function, and even the loss of ageing wrinkles. Although, theoretically, such effects should be possible, further proof is needed to be more convincing.

At the Pacific University of Hawaii on Maui, Gregory Morgan, Ph.D., states that bi-energetic potentials were measured highest in Tachyon water (over any other water ever tested in his laboratory). The Tachyon Energy Research Company at 170 South Beverly Drive, Suite 303, Beverly Hills, California 90212, provides information of their products which cite anecdotal examples and gives, as references, the following:

1. GERBER, Richard. VIBRATIONAL MEDICINE. (Santa Fe, New Mexico: Bear & Co., 1988), p. 147.

2. DAVIDSON, John. SUBTLE ENERGY. (Saffron

123

Walden, Essex, England: C.W. Daniel Co., Ltd., 1987), pp. 202 & 203.

3. FELDMAN, L. "Short bibliography on faster-than-light particles (tachyons)", AMERICAN JOURNAL OF PHYSICS, vol. 42 (March 1974).

4. Op. cit. Davidson pp. 141-145.

5. DAVIDSON, John. THE SECRET OF THE CREATIVE VACUUM. (Saffron Walden, Essex, England: C.W. Daniel Co., Ltd., 1989, pp. 121 & 122.)

****

Chapter 10

Energy Of A Different Kind?

Psycho-Neuro-Immunology (PNI)

The new field of PNI goes a giant step beyond the simple and vague concept that psychotherapy can be useful in treating physical disease. Actually, PNI is a complex of disciplines which have demonstrated that there is no division between what we call mind and body. The information gleaned from the remarkable advances in immunology, neurology, biochemistry, physiology and psychology adds up to an impressive case against any physician, who is not utilizing the "holistic" approach of body, mind and spirit. It is now proven that the brain communicates with the rest of the body, not only by nerves, but by chemical and electromagnetic messengers that travel with cells and fluids.

A single cell, which we have classically thought of as a minute part of the whole, is, in reality, a world unto itself. It mimics, in so many ways, the whole of which it is a part. It becomes obvious that the chemistry produced anywhere under any circumstance, in any part of the body, must and does have a reverberating effect and an almost infinite number of reactions, involving everything that goes on in the human. Carried a step further, because the human is a part of its environment, the same kind of interaction, therefore, goes on between the human and its universe - **And, it is a two-way street!**

All this leaves major questions unanswered. What kind of energy is thought? How does the brain (matter) create this energy? How does the body read this energy and respond? Perhaps PNI should have been included in the chapter on electromagnetics. My guess is that quantum physics is the most rational approach. Its vibrational! How are your vibes?

For thousands of years, it has been known that stress plays an important role in disease, including cancer. However, it has been belittled and ignored by most physicians. Studies have indicated that a patient who does not submit to a dictatorial physician, is more likely to survive. Carl Simonton and Bernie Sigel are the two most well-known physicians, who have sparked both interest and action in demonstrating that patients must take a significant responsibility for their own recovery. Considering the record of medicine in the treatment of cancer, and having learned over several decades that natural methods are far superior to almost anything that medicine has produced, I would conclude that the patient has to be, at least, 90% responsible and the physician, 10% or less.

The role of life purpose and the interaction of the individual in society, has been demonstrated by D. Spiegel and published in the Journal of Mind-Body Health, 1981. Individuals taking part in **group discussion and support**, survive twice as long as those individuals not partaking of this natural "medicine". A fascinating aspect of the study was that mood or attitude did not appear to have any relationship to survival. However, the number of individuals in the group and the fact of participation, seemed to be the determining factors. It makes you pause and wonder, maybe there is something to electromagnetic fields, "auras", and "vibes". Too bad, we don't spend more money on the research of humans in Society, rather than mice in laboratory cages.

The number of concepts, methods, techniques and programs that have to be placed in this category (PNI) is staggering. It would take an encyclopedia to catalogue and describe them all just briefly. Some may argue that some of the items I am including in the list below, i.e. unknown energy fields, faith healing, religion etc. belong elsewhere. They may, in fact, be right. But until they are better understood, I'd rather not label them and wait for future historians to do it with better evidence.

**Hypnosis   Meditation   Transcendental Meditation   Reiki
Yoga   Tai Chi   Touch Healing   Crystal Therapy
Color Therapy   Aroma Therapy   Reflexology   Iridology
Psychic Healing   Voodoo and so on........**

Whatever the final understanding may be, the past arrogant attitudes and blunders of the establishment remind me to be humble, keep an open mind and not to pass judgement until the truth be surely known with proof.

Meanwhile, if it is safe - If it works, - use it!

****

Chapter 11

Suggested Nutritional Supplements...
Algae

SPIRULINA

There are three major forms of algae (there are millions of species). One is from the sea and the others come from fresh water lakes and brackish water. Approximately fifteen years ago, **Spirulina** became popular as a food for losing weight, when included in a diet. In 1982 I did the world's first double-blind study on the use of Spirulina in a diet program. It proved to be effective. In the course of preparing for this study, I reviewed a large volume of literature that had been printed about **Spirulina**. Most notably, was a World Health Organization report outlining the composition of this algae and in which stated that it was the world's richest source of plant protein. Its very unusual amino acid composition is exceptional, not only amongst plants, but it does not appear in animal tissue. It has been recommended by WHO as the most likely solution, to the need for providing a source of protein for the world's hungry.

Wide varieties exist and are often divided by their color, i.e. **green algae, blue algae, blue-green algae, and brown algae**. They uniformly are a rich source of Beta-Carotene which is noted for its anti-oxidant activity and, therefore, for their ability to inhibit cancer growth.

CHLORELLA

Chlorella has been investigated more than any other algae. F. Konishi, S. Matsueda, N. A. Firsova and Y. Miyazawa have all written scientific papers on the anti-tumor activity of chlorella, particularly in **breast cancer** and **leukemia.**

J. Schwartz and G. Shklar utilized Spirulina and Dunaliella in their experiments on hamsters and demonstrated truly remarkable anti-cancer activity.

****

BUGULA

Bugula neretina, an ocean invertebrate, is a plant-like species, which grows under water. They contain bryostatins which have been shown to stimulate immunity.

Leukemia in mice and in humans has been effectively inhibited by this chemical (R. Eckert, Exp Clin Endocrinol, 1990, N. Lilley, Cancer Research, 1990, and R.J. Jones, Blood, 1990).

Bryostatin, derived from bugula, has been used with two other chemotherapeutic substances, TPA and ara-C, in promising laboratory experiments with cancer cells (J.E. Nutt, British Journal of Cancer 1991 and S. Grant, Biochemical Pharmacology, 1991).

****

AMINO ACIDS

ARGININE

Arginine is one of the essential amino acids of the body which comprises the 20% of the amino acids that the body cannot manufacture. Amino acids are the building blocks of proteins, enzymes and hormones. This amino acid is found in milk, eggs, meat, almonds and pistachios, in moderate amounts. Research has revealed that arginine in important in maintaining a healthy immune system, the metabolism of growth hormones, fertility, formation of muscle, the production of collagen and detoxification.

J. Weissburger, in an article written for Toxicology and Applied Pharmacology in 1969, demonstrated that arginine could inhibit **liver cancer** in rats. This finding was confirmed by National Cancer Institute Scientists in 1980 and Japanese scientists in 1985.

J. Reynolds (Annals of Surgery, 1990) demonstrated that arginine increased survival time by its effect on the T-cell response to tumors. Arginine has also been shown to increase natural killer cell activity and to work in conjunction with Lentinan in boosting the immune system (M. Akimoto, 1986).

****

BEE POLLEN

It has been demonstrated that bee pollen is a complete source of nutrition for humans. One of the reasons you have not heard much about it is because it cannot be synthesized and therefore does not get the usual publicity that is given to food substances, supplements and drugs that can be manufactured. Investigators have indicated that there is a special property to pollen that is collected by bees as opposed to the pollen that is collected mechanically from plants.

E. A. Ericsson from the University of Wisconsin, has demonstrated that there is a change in electrical charge in bees carrying pollen. Researchers indicate that the Queen Bee, fed a diet of royal jelly, becomes far superior to the ordinary Worker Bee, as well as having a remarkably extended lifetime.

N.V. Tsitsin, of Russia, in studying the life habits of individuals of the Caucasus region that lived 125 years or more, found that they ate pure bee pollen from bee hives as one of their food staples. If you decide to add bee pollen to your diet, **make sure that you are using bee pollen or royal jelly and not flower pollen.**

The effect on longevity was confirmed by N. P. Yoirich of the Soviet Academy. Other scientists in the Soviet Union, Yugoslavia and in France, support these findings.

W. Robinson reported that bee pollen contained an

anti-carcinogenic substance which slowed the growth of breast tumors (Journal of the National Cancer Institute, 1948).

P. Hernuss of the University of Indiana, advocated the use of bee pollen during radiation therapy for cancer, as it decreased many of the severe side effects. The source of bee pollen is very important for the pollen to be fully enzymatically active. There are very few places in the world where the flowers are free of fertilizers and insecticides. It is also important that the pollen has not been processed or treated with dangerous chemicals. Excessive heating destroys many of the active ingredients.

****

BENZALDEHYDE

The oil of bitter almond is chemically known as, Benzaldehyde. It occurs in apricot kernels and many other foods. In small doses, it is generally regarded as safe. It has been a part of Chinese herbal medicine for centuries. Its role and method of action in cancer therapy is more completely explained in the discussion on Amygdalin (Laetrile).

Dr. N. Kochi reported a dramatic response in sixty-five patients with **inoperable cancers** and reported it in the National Cancer Institute's Cancer Treatment Reports in 1985.

Most studies have not reported toxicity and, even derivatives tested by T. Tatsumura, and reported in the British Journal of Cancer in 1990, proved effective and non-toxic.

E.O. Pettersen in Anti-Cancer Research 1991, reported that a compound created from ascorbic acid (Vitamin C) and Benzaldehyde, destroyed 99% of cancer cells without toxicity.

N. F. McCarty in Medical Hypotheses, 1982, recommended combining Benzaldehyde, Beta-Carotene and antineoplastons as a therapy that could reverse cancer cells to normal without harm to patients (This therapy has my vote, except that I would be more inclined to use Amygdalin).

N. N. Wick and G. B. Fitzgerald in The Journal of Pharmacalogical Science, 1987, demonstrated that Benzaldehyde based drugs were effective against **leukemia,** with **a** significant increase in life expectancy.

Y. Kuroki showed that a Benzaldehyde compound inhibited **lung metastases** in mice (J Cancer Res Clin Oncol 1991).

Research has indicated that natural killer cell activity and Interleukin-2 could be enhanced by benzaldehyde compounds, and that it could also be used in conjunction with chemotherapy (E. Kano, 1986, and K. Masuyama, 1987).

A few reports have appeared which have belittled the effects of benzaldehyde. Their significance must be questioned for the usual reasons that comprise the hallmark of "establishment" studies i.e. they don't use the right substance, they cut the experiment short and distort, diminish or mistate the findings. In this instance they used figs as a source of benzaldehyde and also discounted small but significant results. However, I am sure they were well compensated.

****

CABBAGE (INDOLES)

Since ancient times, cabbage has been eaten for its therapeutic effects. There is no question that this vegetable, along with others of the cruciferous species, i.e. brussel sprouts, cauliflower and broccoli, contain indoles.

Indoles have been shown experimentally to be effective in the prevention of **breast, stomach and colon cancer**. It is also protective against radiation (P.N. Albert, J. Ethnopharmacol. 1983; G. S. Stoewsand, 1988; and J. J. Michnovicz, J Natl. Cancer Inst.1990).

Broccoli, kale, cauliflower and brussel sprouts contain another substance, Sulphoraphane, which exhibits very strong anti-cancer effects. U. Zhang, et al., and H.J. Prochaska, presented this information to the proceedings of the National Academy of Sciences (U.S.A.) 1992. Expert opinion is overwhelming toward their inclusion in the family diet.

****

CANTHAXANTHIN

This food coloring agent has been primarily used medically as protection against the damaging effects from exposure to sunlight. The evidence that it is also an immune booster is supported by many researchers (A.P. Gupta, et al., Int J Dermatol. 1985; A. Bendich, and S.S. Shapiro, Journal of Nutrition, 1986; B.S. Alan, Nutr Cancer. 1988; S.T. Mayne, Nutr. Cancer. 1989; A. Pung, Carcinogenesis, 1988, J. Schwartz, Nutr. Cancer, 1988). The fact that Canthaxanthin is not converted into vitamin A, indicates that it must work through some other effect. The various studies sited have indicated the following activities and abilities of Canthaxanthin:

1. Enhances vitamin E in tissues.
2. Acts as an anti-oxidant.
3. Effective against chemically induced cancers in mice by inhibiting growth.
4. Inhibits growth of salivary gland tumors in rats.
5. Local injection causes regression of tumors.
6. Reduces incidence of mammary cancers in mice.

Canthaxanthin has been known to cause changes in the retina, mainly by discoloration. However, it is well established these effects are reversible (C. Harnois, Archives of Ophthalmology, 1988 and 1989; N.N. Nijman, 1989; H. Leyon, Acta Ophthalmol, Copenhagen, 1990).

Because of **one** case of aplastic anemia in a woman who had taken Canthaxanthin for tanning purposes, the AMA has warned of its use (JAMA, 1990).

It should be noted that Canthaxanthin is a natural food additive and is present in many products throughout the world. It is unquestionably effective against cancer, when combined with Beta-Carotene and Vitamin A.

****

CHLOROPHYLL

Chlorophyll is responsible for the green color of plants and plays a vital roll in photosynthesis, which is the process by which light is converted into plant energy. Chlorophyll is an effective anti-cancer substance. It protects against many environmental mutagens including cigarette smoke, nitrates, coal dust, diesel omissions and many others (C.N. Lai, Mutation Research, 1980; R. Turwell, Mutation Research, 1985; T. Ong, Mutation Research, 1986).

Its action is mainly as an anti-oxidant and is extremely effective in neutralizing free radicals. Experiments in rats fed chlorophyll, show fewer carcinogenic changes in the cells of their colon (E. Robbins and R. Nelson, Anti-Cancer Research, 1989).

Chlorophyll has shown an ability to protect fruit flies from the effects of radiation (S. Zimmering, Mutation Research, 1990).

Anti-cancer abilities have been confirmed by H.W. Renner, Mutation Research, 1990; and J.R. Warner, et al., Mutation Research, 1991).

****

DHEA (DEHYDROEPIANDROSTERONE)

DHEA is classified as a hormone and is the second most abundant steroid produced in the body. Cholesterol is the most abundant. It is secreted by the adrenal glands and very little is known about its function. The production of DHEA declines markedly with age to a level of 5% in the very old when compared to the young.

In 1981, A.G. Schwartz in an article in Nutrition and Cancer explained in detail the complicated role DHEA played in inhibiting the development of cancer. He noted that cancer causing substances (carcinogens) required metabolic activation by oxidative enzymes to cause cancer. DHEA inhibits this process by lowering the levels of these oxidases. The decline in DHEA production parallels a rise in the incidence of cancer, obesity and heart disease.

The inhibitory role of DHEA in the synthesis of fatty acids in the body is similar to the theoretical model described for cancer. It is important not to confuse these fatty acids with the essential fatty acids, those not produced by the body (see the very important discussion in the chapter on linseed oil).

These theories have been tested in the laboratory. T. Yen et al., in Lipids, 1977, demonstrated that DHEA PREVENTED THE DEVELOPMENT OF OBESITY in rats, in spite of the fact that the rats were genetically destined to become obese (I mention this because I know how many people struggle with trying to stay slim or lose weight.). The rats also displayed youthful vitality and had a **much lower risk of cancer,** even though genetically they were coded to develop specific cancers. In addition, their **life span was extended by 50%.**

Supportive evidence for these hypotheses is provided by D.Y. Wang et al., in their article on the low level of DHEA in the blood of women with **breast cancer** (European Journal of Cancer, 10, 1974) and similar findings by R.D. Bulbrook (Lancet 2, 1971).

J.W. Nyce et al., inhibited the development of induced **colon cancers** in mice with DHEA (Carcinogenesis, 1984)

A. G. Schwatz et al., inhibited induced **lung cancer** development in mice (Carcinogenesis, 1981)

L.L. Pashko et al., inhibited DNA synthesis of **skin and breast** tissue with DHEA (Carcinogenesis, 1981)

DHEA is non-toxic and legal to use, but may require a prescription depending on your country of residence. The resource section directs your physician as to where to obtain it.

****

ESSENTIAL FATTY ACIDS

(See the chapter on linseed oil for extensive information on fatty acid metabolism.)

****

FISH OILS

Many studies have established that the high intake of fish oil is related to a low incidence of **cancers of the breast, colon and pancreas.** The Omega-3 group of fatty acids are the main compounds of fish oil. Their role as a treatment in arthritis and heart disease is becoming more widely accepted.

L. Kaizer in Nutrition and Cancer, 1989, stated that the more fish that people included in their diet, the less **breast cancer** they were likely to develop.

H. Gabor, et al., slowed down the growth of transplanted breast tumors in mice by feeding them fish oil.

N. Tisdale and J.K. Dhesi reported in Cancer Research 1990, that fish **oils were as effective against cancer as the chemotherapeutic drugs**, Cyclophosphamide and 5-FU, without any of the toxicity and at much lesser cost.

M. Sakaguchi, N.A. Lindner, and B.S. Reddy have all demonstrated the beneficial roll of fish oils in the prevention of **colon cancer.**

The use of fish oils, therapeutically, reduces the level of cholesterol and triglycerides in the blood. J. Dyerberg and H.O. Bang discovered that a diet, very rich in fish oils (high fat diet) actually lowered the instance of cardiovascular disease. This was found to be true in the Eskimo population, where the cold water variety of fish was ingested. The Omega-3 fatty acids, of which this oil consists, appear to be the important ingredients. These oils are in the polyunsaturate fatty acid group. The people of Scandinavia also benefit in the same way, from this type of diet.

In 1985, D. Kronhout, published an article in the New England Journal of Medicine, in which he showed that the risk of cardiovascular disease was reduced to one third in those men who ate between 32-144 grams of fish a day, as compared to men eating only 1-14 grams on an average.

M. Davidson, in an article also published in the New England Journal of Medicine, showed that taking fish oil capsules reduced cholesterol levels by 24% and triglyceride levels by 48%.

R.A. Karmali, of Rutgers University, performed studies on animals which indicated that the Omega-3 fatty acids could protect against **breast and prostate cancer.** Other studies have also shown that it may be preventive in **colon and lung cancer.**

The beneficial effects of Omega-3 fatty acids have been confirmed by W.E. Connor of the Amaan Health Services University, J.N. Kramer of Albany Medical College and W. Lands of the University of Illinois. As it now stands, there is substantial evidence that the Omega-3 fatty acid is playing an important role in the prevention or treatment of rheumatoid arthritis, cirrhosis and cancer.

Studies also indicate that the fatty acids are important for the acceptance of surgical grafts and in the development of brain and nerve tissue. N. Neuringer and W.E. Connor have done studies which indicate the importance of the presence of these acids in the development of brain and retinal tissue, during the fetal stage of development and infancy.

****

VEGETABLE SOURCES

There are vegetable sources of the Omega-3 fatty acids and they include the herb, purslane. The importance of the role of the essential fatty acids began 150 years ago, with the work of Professor B. J. van Liebig. Many scientists have published literally thousands of papers on this subject and in 1920, the Nobel prize in Physiology and Medicine was won by Dr. Otto Meyerhof, who demonstrated the role of linoleic acid and sulphur proteins in the oxygenation of tissue. In the eleven years that followed, two more Nobel prizes were won by Albert Szent-Gyorgy and Dr. Otto Warburg in 1931. Both related to the role of fatty acids, oxygenation of tissue and the development of cancer. Butter and cream contain trace amounts of fatty acids. Linseed oil and cottage cheese, however, contain far greater amounts and are certainly a far more beneficial way of securing these important food substances.

****

EVENING PRIMROSE OIL

Evening Primrose oil is an excellent source of gamma-linolenic acid (GLA). Elsewhere in this book the roll of this fatty acid is discussed at length in relation to linseed oil, another excellent source of fatty acids. Evidence exists that GLA can normalize malignant cells and even reverse their growth. The work of David F. Horrobin (Medical Hypotheses, 1980) is supported by researchers, C van der Merwe, F. Fujiwara, N.

Dippenaar, Y. Haiashi, M.E. Begin, S. Ikushima, W.P. Leary, J.H. Botha, J. Booyens, L. Koenig, U. N. Das, N.S. Gardener, J.R. Duncan and C.S. Cunnane. The papers produced by these various investigators show that GLA is effective against **bladder cancer, melanomas, breast, lung, prostate and nerve tissue cancers.**

****

FIBER

In the 1960's Denis Burkitt studied the effect of the fiber-rich diet of Africans on the very low incidence of colon cancer. In 1978, he published a landmark article in the American Journal of Clinical Nutrition which indicated the important roll of fiber in the prevention of colon cancer. With the increase of commercially produced low fiber foods, the incidence of colon cancer has increased from rare to common. The advice given by physicians, who advocated dietary measures in the prevention and treatment of disease, was, for many years, looked upon as quackery. However, Dr. Burkitt, who was extremely famous, could not be ignored.

Fiber works through the following pathways:
1. Absorption and elimination of carcinogenic substances (S.A. Bingham, Proc Nutr Soc. 1990).
2. Facilitation and elimination of excess estrogen (D.J. Pusateri, American Journal of Clinical Nutrition, 1990).
3. Conversion of bile acids that can damage DNA (P.Y. Cheha and H. Burnstein, Nutr. Cancer. 1990).

Different sources of fiber have different effects. Rice bran was found to stimulate the immune system and, in mice, was effective against carcinomas (E. Ito, 1985).

Bran proved to be effective against drug-induced **colon cancer** (W.F. Chen and H.S. Goldsmith, 1978).

Psylliun husks proved to inhibit the ability of a carcinogenic agent, DMH, which causes colon cancer (J. Roberts-Andersen, Nutr Cancer. 1987).

Wheat bran was also effective in combatting **colon cancer**

(K. Watanabe, J Nat'l Cancer Inst. 1979).

The American Cancer Society, the U.S. National Research Council Committee on Diet, Nutrition and Cancer, the National Cancer Institute of Canada, Harvard Medical School, the Wistar Institute in Philadelphia and many other investigators have confirmed that dietary fiber is exceptionally important in prevention of cancer, however, an improvement in the entire diet plays an essential role.

Associated with a low fiber intake and the high incidence of breast cancer, is high animal fat intake and low vitamin C intake (G.R. Howe, J Nat'l Cancer Inst. 1990; S. Shankar, Hematol Oncol Clin North Am. 1991; W.C. Willett, N Engl J Med. 1990; P. Van t'Veer, Int J Cancer. 1990).

The incidence of colon cancer amongst the Japanese is very low. In spite of the fact that the fiber intake is approximately the same as the diet in the USA, the Japanese consume half the amount of fat. It would appear that a combination of low fat and high fiber provides protection against this form of cancer. Actually it provides **ten times** the protection!

****

HERBS

NOTE: THE USE OF HERBS IS NOT RECOGNIZED BY THE FDA OR THE MEDICAL ESTABLISHMENT. MANY HERBS ARE USED BY HERBALISTS, NATUROPATHS, AND OTHER PRACTITIONERS IN MANY STATES. HOWEVER, THEY ARE GENERALLY NOT ALLOWED TO MAKE ANY CLAIMS IN REFERENCE TO THEIR USE. THE INFORMATION PROVIDED IN THIS CHAPTER IS FOR THE ENLIGHTENMENT OF THE READER AND IS **NOT TO BE CONSIDERED AS ADVICE OR RECOM-MENDATIONS OF A MEDICAL NATURE.** MY OPINION, HOWEVER, IS THAT THEY ARE SUPERIOR, 95% OF THE TIME, TO ANY PHARMACEUTICAL DRUG!

The role of herbs and herbal mixtures in medicine dates back thousands of years. Their use is well documented in the hundreds of books published in the last century alone. If a medical claim is made for them by a company, the FDA usually steps in and confiscates the product. The First Amendment (free speech) allows a book or a periodical to write about their use, but a company cannot provide the same information on the label or in literature which is in any way associated with the company. This also applies to vitamins, minerals and other supplements. As I write, most herbs are still available in many herbal shops and health food stores.

Physicians of medicine, with a few exceptions, know nothing of the use of herbs in the prevention and treatment of disease. Many aren't even aware that digitalis is an herb. Its use in modern medicine exists only because of the curiosity and diligent testing by of a young physician centuries ago. Pharmaceutical companies produced it and then extracted its "active" ingredients in order to obtain a patent. The reason given, of course, is that they wanted to provide a more potent product and one in which the dosage could be more accurately controlled. This is true only in part. The power and toxicity of digitoxin, digoxin, etc., are well known to every physician. Older physicians, most of whom are dead or no longer in practice, felt more comfortable in the safety of the original digitalis leaf. Younger physicians coming into practice in the 50's had no means for comparison and were being taught pharmacology with emphasis on the newer preparations while in medical school. In reality, the influence of pharmaceutical detail persons (salespersons) has a significant impact on the busy physician who often foolishly believes that they are truly knowledgeable enough to provide a quick educational summary on the product. This is rarely true. These representatives are frequently misinformed by their companies and instructed to stress the "good" points and leave out the bad.

The record of pharmaceutical companies on drug recalls and claim revisions is witness to the dishonesty of the industry and to the flaws and ill-placed dependency on what is obviously and incorrectly referred to as the "scientific" method of proof. A basic error in the current scientific approach to therapeutics is the belief that the individual components of biological phenomenon are sufficient to explain the whole phenomenon itself. This might indeed be true if we actually:

✦ had **all** the parts;

✦ understood their **inter-relationship** completely,

✛ comprehended the **synergism** involved in the complex inter-reactions and their ultimate effects on the whole;
✛ realized fully the changes occurring constantly because of the effects of time, intensity, thought, emotions and the infinite kinds of variations in the internal and external environment of that whole.

Put simply, biochemical-Pharmaceutical science today arrogantly and ignorantly formulates an indelible, immovable position which they call scientific fact and proof, and then is forced to explain failure on the basis of "side-effects, "complications" or the "patient failed to respond" - and then they settle for the "lesser of two evils" or a drug recall!

An incredible example of this tragic folly is the unfolding of the current AIDS scam. In this instance, the AIDS hypothesis has named an innocuous virus, that is present everywhere and has been around for centuries (we have become aware of its presence because of new instruments and techniques), the "AIDS" virus without a single shred of scientific evidence that it causes AIDS or transmits any of the diseases attributed to it. The causes of AIDS, as it is now called, have been known for at least sixty years. But that is the subject of another book I have just completed called *"The Ultimate Deception"*. It is an astounding and unbelievably shocking expose based on scientific fact and **proven by scientific documentation**.

While modern drugs, which have contributed little good and much harm to patients, are widely used and touted as "wonders", herbs which have stood the test of time are largely ignored. However, it is not my intention to write another book on herbs. This chapter will deal only with herbal formulas that are currently considered useful in cancer. Keep in mind, if you decide to investigate herbs further for this purpose, that herbs which "detoxify" or boost the body's defenses are the ones most likely to be applicable.

There is a concern, that imported herbs are exposed to irradiation and gassing by government agencies of some countries which can alter their properties and even render them potentially harmful. The effects of irradiation or gassing on any food has not been fully investigated and is being challenged by professional and citizen groups. I have been told that the most reliable sources are local reputable growers. I have chosen to mention herb formulas that have interesting, but sometimes sparsely documented, histories of use. The information has been gathered from books and individuals, some of whom market the products, and from people who are using them. Because most patients I have talked to, have been on therapeutic programs of one form or another, it is impossible to be able to attribute their successes to a specific remedy. I have heard many stories from apparently sincere individuals, who "know people" who have taken one treatment or another, and whose cancers have disappeared and were confirmed by medical examination and tests. It is in this frame-work that I am presenting a few of the most popular herbal preparations.

Herbs, which are simply plants, have been used throughout recorded history and evidence exists for their successful treatment of disease. Herbal medicine has been practiced by every major world civilization. Approximately half of all modern pharmaceuticals are derived from herbs. Animals naturally seek out certain herbs in the self-treatment of disease. This would indicate that man learned from animals and therefore places the beginnings of herbal medicine to a time many millions of years ago. Simple observation of primitive, inexpensive herbal treatments, as compared to the expensive and toxic pharmaceutical derivations, reveals that we would be far better off to go back in time and avoid the disaster of the modern pharmaceutical industry. Modern medicines are a classical example of "paying through the nose" in order to get "shafted".

****

ALOE

The aloe plant has become the basic ingredient of a large number of commercial preparations in the form of creams, lotions, gels and shampoos. The juice of the aloe is being used for cleansing of the colon and intestinal problems. Toxicity and side effects are relatively rare and not usually severe. Almost every conceivable benefit has been claimed for aloe over the centuries - most of them justified.

Because it is a plant, chemical analysis has revealed a host of substances, one of which has been shown in mice to have anti-leukemic activity (S.N. Kupchan, 1976).

The anti-cancer activity of aloe indicate that its action is through stimulation of the scavenging white blood cells of the immune system (L. Ralamboranto, Archives of the Pasteur Institute, 1982).

The many studies carried out by Russian scientists, have done more to establish a respectable place in modern medicine for aloe than any other group of investigators. N.V. Gribel and V.G. Pashinskii, in Vopr Onkol. 1986, showed that aloe juice **reduced tumor** mass and the frequency of metastases in rats.

R. Berkow in the Merck Manual, wrote of aloe's ability to protect individuals with weakened immune systems against infection.

S. Solar, publishing in the Archives of the Pasteur Institute in 1980, showed that aloe could prevent infection in mice, if used several days before exposure.

J.Y. Brossat and his group, in the same journal the following year, demonstrated that aloe was effective in preventing serious infections from bacteria, parasites and even fungus. These studies give great credence to those individuals who drink aloe on a daily basis, as a protective against disease.

Y. Sato wrote of aloe's protective effect on the skin against X-rays and K. Saki demonstrated its protection of the liver, particularly against alcohol. All of this evidence makes aloe a logical choice in health maintenance and, in particular, as a cancer preventative because of its obvious protection and benefits to the immune system.

****

ASTRAGALUS

Astragalus was known in the Wild, Wild West of America, as the "locoweed". There is no question that astragalus is an extraordinary booster of the immune system and is so recognized by Science. In spite of this, if you ask your doctor about it, he would probably think you were talking about asparagus and then give you a weird glance.

D.T. Chu in the Journal of Clinical Laboratory Immunology,

1988, demonstrated its use in **cancer** and J. Jaing, in 1986, showed that astragalus protected the liver of animals against the toxic effects of the common cleaning fluid, carbon tetrachloride. It has also been used to protect the liver in patients receiving chemotherapy (Z.L. Zhang, Journal of Ethnopharmacology, 1990).

Naturally, as one might expect, chemicals derived from this inexpensive weed, have been tested successfully in preventing the spread of metastases, of **melanoma** to the lungs in mice. M.J. Humphries reported the effect of this chemical "swainsonine" in Cancer Research in 1988 and J.W. Dennis confirmed its action in Cancer Research in 1990.

S. A. Newton, et al., reported on the protective effects of swainsonine on the **bone marrow** during chemotherapy. My suggestion is to get "locoweed" and use it until scientists prove that they can do a safer and better job than nature. That means, science will do better, when "hell freezes over".

****

MISTLETOE

A commercial preparation of fermented mistletoe, known as **Iscador,** is widely marketed in Europe and its use has extended to some degree throughout the world. Most research has been conducted in Germany. Mistletoe is a folk remedy that has been advocated since the 1920's, as a therapy for cancer. It has been rejected by the American Cancer Society - of course!

It is believed that a lectin labelled ML-1, and which is a plant protein, **stimulates the immune system** by increasing white blood cells, particularly the macrophages and natural killer cells. It also increase thymus activity, thus resulting in an increased immune response (T. Hojto, et al., Cancer Research 1989; and R. Rentea, Lab Investigations 1981)

Iscador has been found effective against lymphoma in mice and in a large study involving more than one hundred and sixty patients with **advanced lung cancer.** These studies not only showed that Iscador stimulated the immune system, It directly destroyed cancer cells and prolonged survival time (G. Salzer, Oncology 1986).

Ovarian cancer responded three times better to Iscador than to standard chemotherapy involving Cytobal (W. Hassauer, et al., Onkologie, 1979). No wonder the American Cancer Society condemned it!

Other studies indicate that Iscador is not effective in kidney cancer and carcinosarcoma. It is important to note that viscumalbum, the European mistletoe, and Phoradendrom flavescens, the American mistletoe, are both potentially poisonous, therefore, commercially prepared compounds are strongly advised over home made concoctions.

****

HERBAL FORMULAS

Herbal mixtures have been formulated to assist the body in situations of stress caused by disease. The following formulas can be used as indicated.

ANTI-ANXIETY (calming effect) Formula:

When confronted by a serious illness such as cancer, it is completely normal to experience the following emotions; anxiety, fear, despondency and isolation. Instead of tranquilizers and antidepressants use this formula.

Formula:
Passion Flower Black Cohosh Root
Ginger Root
Hops (Oil - humulene, myrcene, B-carophyllene, farnescene)
Skullcap
Wood Betony
Valerian Root

Preparation: 400 mg. blend per capsule

Dosage: 1-3 capsules, two to four times daily

Contraindications: Usually not taken with prescription medication unless separated by 3 to 4 hours. If sensitive to estrogen, take with caution.

****

GLANDULAR AND NERVE TONIC:

Improves ability to detoxify. It is used as a general tonic and acts as a pain reliever, anti-spasmodic, anti-inflammatory and wound healer with antibiotic properties

Formula:
> Blue Vervain (Verbena hastata)
> Cayenne (Capsicum annuum)
> Chamomile Flowers (Matricaria chamomilla)
> Dandelion Root (Taraxacum officinale)
> Gentian Root (Gentiana lutea)
> Goldenseal Root (Hydrastis canadensis)
> Kelp (Laminaria, Macrocystis, Ascophyllum)
> Saw Palmetto Berries (Serenoa repens-sabal)
> Skullcap, (Scutellaria lateriflora)
> Wood Betony (Stachys officinalis, Pedicularis canadensis)
> Yellow Dock Root (Rumex crispus)

Preparation: 450 mg. blend per capsule

Dosage: 2-3 capsules per day (take with meals)

****

CANCER, TOXICITY AND POISONING:

Heavy metal poisoning. Contamination of water air and food. Radiation of all types. In view of the fact that these contaminants are carcinogenic, it is recommended for individuals with cancer and for those who have had chemotherapy or radiation.

Formula:
> Alfalfa (Medicago sativa)
> Algin (algae and seaweeds)
> Apple Pectin
> Kelp (Laminaria, Macrocystis, Ascophyllum)

Preparation: 450 mg. blend per capsule

Dosage: 4 capsules per day (taken with meals)

> **Contraindications:** May deplete trace elements, therefore replace - particularly zinc and manganese. If diarrhea occurs, reduce dosage and take 1/2 teaspoon of cornstarch with 2 slippery elm capsules.

****

RECOVERY FORMULA:

Useful after serious illness or surgery.
> Buckthorn Bark (Rhamnus frangula)
> Burdock Root (Arctium lappa)
> Cascara Sagrada Bark (Rhamnus purshinana)
> Chaparral (Larrea divaricata)
> Kelp (Laminaria, Macrocystis, Ascophyllum)
> Licorice Root (Glycyrrhiza glabra)
> Oregon Grape Root (Mahonia aquifolium)
> Prickly Ash Bark (Zanthoxylum americanum)
> Red Clover (Trifolium pratense)
> Sarsaparilla Root (Smilax Officinalis, Smilax aristolochi aceafolia)
> Stillingia (Stillingia sylvatica

Preparation: 350 mg. blend per capsule

Dosage: 8-10 capsules per day in two to three doses.

Drink plenty of water!

> **Contraindications:** Do not take with prescription drugs,

particularly chemotherapy, cortisone or sulfa drugs. If unavoidable, separate by three hours.

****

AYURVEDIC HERBAL MEDICINE

One of my favorite medical writers is Deepak Chopra, M.D. He has written wonderful, popular books on the combining of Indian medical traditions and modern Western science. Various letters and articles appeared in The Journal of the American Medical Association (JAMA) in 1991, which were obviously printed because of the impressive content. When the editors finally woke up to its great popularity and possible impact on their monopoly of allopathic medicine, they tried to detract from the historical intelligence of these writings by attacking it as a "marketing scheme", and even denounced it as a hoax. So much for the integrity and purpose of American medicine's "banner journal". For your edification, I will summarize the information.

Ayurvedic medicine has many principles and techniques in common with Chinese medicine and with almost all schools of natural thought and practice. The articles in JAMA involved a discussion of two herbal compounds, M4 and M5 which were found to effectively reduce the incidence of **breast cancer** that was chemically induced in laboratory animals. These compounds were also effective in treating **breast cancer**. Studies done on lung cancer, metastases with M4, were also successful and a common brain tumor, **neuroblastoma**, was normalized by M5. These herbal compounds contained antioxidants which explains their anti-carcinogenic activity.

****

CANNABIS

Cannabis, also known as Marijuana, is the best known of all herbs. Although every sin on the face of the earth has been blamed on its use, A.E. Munson, et al., in the Journal of the National Cancer Institute in 1975, wrote of the anti-neoplastic activity of marijuana derivatives. To the amazement of all readers, it described the retarding effect on the growth of **lung cancer** in mice, in as little as ten days and even more pronounced beneficial effects, with continued use.

Marijuana has also been used by cancer patients to counteract the nausea and vomiting caused by chemotherapy (P. V. Tortorice, Pharmacotherapy, 1990; H.J. Eyre, Cancer, 1984).

To make sure that patients with cancer would not enjoy the usual effects known for marijuana, science has spared them this asocial benefit by testing synthetic substances (dronabinol and nabilone - N. Lane, American Journal of Clinical Oncology, 1990), which, of course, will undoubtedly have "side-effects" at an exorbitant price. Then, it will obviously be socially acceptable!

A.M. Dalzell in the Archives of the Diseases of Children, 1986, honestly pointed out that Nabilone had a higher incidence of side effects than occurred when smoking marijuana!

****

CHAPARRAL

This common shrub of the American South-West, is usually prepared in the form of a tea. As expected, the pharmaceutical industry is again trying to out-do nature by exploring the anti-cancer properties of what they refer to as the "active ingredient", Nordihydroguaiaretic acid (NDGA).

Chaparral is commonly referred to as the creosote bush. NDGA was shown by S. Birkenfeld to reduce the occurrence of **colon cancer** in rats, fed a chemical that induced that cancer.

D.K. Shalini demonstrated NDGA's ability to protect genes **against carcinogens** and published this experiment in Molecular Cell Biochemistry, 1990.

The **breast cancer** preventive effect of NDGA was demonstrated by D.L. McCormick and A.M. Spicer (Cancer Lett. 1987).

Leukemia cell cultures were inhibited by NDGA (A.M. Miller, Journal of Laboratory Clinical Medicine, 1989) and human **brain cancer** cell growth were likewise inhibited by NDGA (D.E. Wilson, Journal of Neurosurgery, 1989).

Cancer cell inhibition was intensively explored in the doctorate thesis of J. Zemora (Auburn University, 1984). 179

Regression of the deadly **melanoma** and treatment of **choriocarcinoma** and **lymphosarcoma** have been sited by C.R. Smart in Cancer Chemotherapy Reports, 1969, and American Cancer Society, 1971.

D. Vanden Berghe demonstrated the anti-cancer and anti-viral activity of other chaparral extracts and P. Train wrote of its use as an anti-bacterial.

Naturally, NDGA is toxic to the kidney and can be deadly when combined with some biologicals (D.R. Shasky, Journal of the American Academy of Dermatology 1986; and J.D. Gardner, Kidney International, 1987).

Because of a rare case in which signs of liver damage showed up after several months of taking chaparral leaf, M. Katz, in the Journal of Clinical Gastroenterology, 1990, warned that "the public and the medical profession must be wary of all 'harmless' non-prescription medications, whether purchased in pharmacies or elsewhere". M. Katz, of course, did not site all the horrendous problems with the synthetic NDGA, of which, I am sure, he approves. Of course, it's acceptable under the supervision of a doctor, it is then professionally managed death. How can we justify the attacks on a Dr. Kavorkian ("Dr. Death") when thousands of doctors do it every day without the patient's informed consent?

****

CHINESE HERBAL MEDICINE

Chinese medicine is based upon intensive and patient observation that has been carried out through more than 4,000 years. From these observations, came philosophical concepts, that have stood the test of time and are being constantly verified by modern scientific discovery. The Western physician, un-aware of the depth of meaning in the Chinese traditional philosophy, looks with disdain at their therapies and perceives them as primitive. The World Health Organization has called for a re-examination of ancient medical traditions and their assimilation into the health systems of each country. This has occurred mostly in countries of Asia and in Mexico and Africa.

The Chinese traditional physicians use a root called **Actinidia**. Its use in inhibiting **liver cancer** growth and other tumors, was discussed in Planta Med. 1989, by G. Franz.

Chemotherapy has been combined with **Rabdosia Rubescens** and has proven to be excellent in combination with chemotherapy (R.L. Wang, 1986).

DNA synthesis is inhibited by **Baohuside - 1**, a natural plant extract, and was, therefore, tested against various cancers by S.Y. Li, Cancer Lett., 1990.

The Chinese have investigated synthetic compounds, similar to extracts from the dried body of the **Chinese Blister Beetle (Mylabris)**. These compounds were demonstrated to be effective against **liver cancer** (G.S. Wang, Journal of Ethnopharmacology, 1989).

The Chinese have been noted for their traditional teas that are used as tonics. **Golden Book Tea** and **Six Flavor Tea** have proved useful in conjunction with chemotherapy and radiation against **lung cancer** (X.Y. Liu and N.Q. Ang, 1990).

Y.B. Ji tested the use of **Bu Zhong Qi Wan**, a pill used to stimulate body energy, along with cyclophosphamide, a chemotherapeutic agent and found that it decreased toxicity and enhanced its anti-cancer activity.

****

GINSENG

The herb, **Eleutherococcus**, is the best species of ginseng. It is rich in vitamins and minerals and has been used for centuries in the Orient for improving brain function and general health, to provide energy, decrease stress and normalize blood pressure. It is believed to slow down the ageing process. This herb, with the scientific name, **Hydrocotylee asiatica**, is obtained from islands in the Indian Ocean. It is believed to have rejuvenating properties and is primarily a stimulant for mental and physical fatigue. Ginseng has gained tremendous popularity, probably because it was touted as a "sexual stimulant" in recent decades. Ginseng is not a single herb. There are actually three plants that are referred to by this one name. It is therefore necessary, when choosing its use, that you get the appropriate herb. Almost every conceivable benefit has been attributed to Ginseng.

Panax Quinquefolius, the American Ginseng, has been shown to revert **cancerous liver cells** to normal (S. Odashima, European Journal of Cancer, 1979; and H. Abe, Experientia, 1979).

Melanoma cells can be reverted to normal by one of the chemicals in Ginseng (T. Ota, Cancer Research, 1987).

Eleutherococcus senticocus, the Siberian Ginseng, boosts the effect of white blood cells and has been used with patients receiving anti-cancer therapy (V.I. Kupin, Vopr Onkol. 1986).

J. P. Kim, in a study using Ginseng and other spices on **cancers of the gastrointestinal tract,** discovered that salt and red pepper encouraged cancer formation. The use of Ginseng during pregnancy has not been thoroughly investigated and, therefore, should be used with considerable caution.

****

THE ESSAIC FORMULA

In recent years, this formula has gained notoriety. There are interesting, substantiated accounts of its recent use in the treatment of cancer. Dr. Gary Glum has investigated and written extensively about the Essaic Formula in his book, ''Calling of An Angel''. The formula became known through the work of Rene Caisse, a nurse who obtained it from a patient who had received it from an Ojibway herbalist. In the early 1920's, Caisse, who lived in Canada, began giving the preparation to any one who requested it as a treatment for cancer. It is reported that even the worst cases were cured or lived longer than expected and were free of pain. As one would expect, the government became involved. More than 55,000 signatures were collected on her behalf, thus allowing her to continue her work. When Caisse died in 1978, the Canadian Ministry of Health and Welfare destroyed all of her documents. (Isn't it amazing that there are so many well-documented cases of the destruction of records of this nature that have occurred in nations where free speech is supposedly protected? ''Book burning" is obviously not just an historical event that happened in Nazi Germany! One has to wonder why democratic countries feel compelled to suppress knowledge of any kind?

The treatment and control of cancer is an immense multi-billion dollar industry. The prevention and cure is not. Dr. Charles Brusch, personal physician to President John F. Kennedy, treated thousands of patients with cancer. Dr. Brusch stated that Essaic was a cure for cancer and was placed under a "gag-order" by the Federal Government. Dr. Brusch treated and cured his own cancer with Essaic and his records are still preserved.

The most important herb in the formula is SHEEP'S SORREL and it is **non-toxic**. This herb is banned in Canada and in the United States. It is, however, an extremely common weed and easily found by anyone who recognizes it. It is not the only herb that has been banned when news of its use in cancer got out. Rene Caisse had been given special permission by the Canadian Government to treat individuals with cancer. As in so many instances of a similar nature, the cases were limited to certified and well-documented terminally ill patients. declared incurable by the establishment. She was not allowed to charge for her services. Many of these hopeless patients lived more than thirty-five years after treatment. Caisse also discovered that the ESSAIC FORMULA was a preventative for many diseases and was effective in correcting thyroid disorders, stomach ulcers and diabetes. Recently it has been used in the treatment of AIDS.

The ESSAIC FORMULA consists of four herbs:
SHEEP'S SORREL (Rumex Acetosella) - 16 ounces in powdered form
BURDOCK ROOT (Arctium Lappa) - 6 1/2 cups in cut form
RUBARB ROOT (Rheum Palmatum) - 1 ounce in powdered form
SLIPPERY ELM BARK (Ulmus Fulva) - 4 ounces in powdered form

PREPARATION:
The dry ingredients are mixed thoroughly.

Place **only one cup** of the dry mixture in 2 gallons of sodium-free distilled water that has been boiling for 30 minutes in a 4 gallon **covered** pot (at sea level - if at higher elevations boil longer).

Store the remainder of the drymixture of herbs in a dark cool area as the herbs are sensitive to light. Stir and continue to boil (covered) for 10 more minutes. Remove the pot from the heat and scrape down the sides of the pot, stir well, cover again with a lid, let stand for 12 hours and then heat quickly to **near** boilingfor 20 minutes, but **DO NOT BOIL.**

Strain the liquid into a 3 gallon pot. Clean the 4 gallon pot and strain the liquid once more back into it. Immediately pour the hot liquid into sterilized bottles through a funnel and cap tightly. When the bottles cool tighten the caps again.

REFRIGERATE. IF A MOLD FORMS - DISCARD! SUPPLIES:

A 3 and a 4 gallon pot with lids, funnel, spatula, fine mesh double strainer - **ALL OF STAINLESS STEEL.** Measuring cup, kitchen scale with ounce measurements and at least 12 or more sterilized amber glass bottles with airtight caps.

BE SURE ALL SUPPLIES ARE STERILIZED BEFORE USE!

DIRECTIONS FOR USE:

As a **preventive**: Shake bottle and take 2 tablespoons (4 oz)of ESSIAC, cold or warmed (not with microwave) at bedtime, but at least 2 hours after eating.
When used as **therapy**, 4 tablespoons are taken twice daily. If the problem is in the stomach, it is advised to dilute the ESSAIC with an equal amount of sodium-free distilled water.

****

UBIQUINONE (Coenzyme Q10)

This substance is present in many foods and can be manufactured by the body. It has been used to protect the heart against the toxic action of anti-cancer drugs (K. Okada, Cancer Research, 1980, E.P. Cortes, Cancer Treat Rep. 1978). Ubiquinone is felt to be of use in times of stress and is, therefore, recommended by many health practitioners for many illnesses, including cancer. It is available in capsules.

****

Chapter 12

Let Your Medicine Be Your Food

(Items To Use In Your Meals)

MUSHROOMS

KOMBUCHA

(Often referred to as "The Champagne of Life" and "The Gift of Life From the Sea". Known in France as the Champion of Longevity and in China as the "Divine Che")

The story about this unusual "tea fungus" probably begins as far back as 221 B.C. with the Tin Dynasty in China. Fungi were considered to be a way of achieving immortality. The fungus was introduced to Japan in 414 A.D. by a Korean physician named Kombu. The benefits reaped by its medical use, earned Kombu the honor of having the fungus named after him. Kombucha tea has enjoyed great popularity in Russia for many centuries.

Dr. Rudolf Sklenar of Germany, in his book, "The Tea Fungus of China" recounts 40 years of remarkable therapeutic success with its use. There are several other books available for further reference, notably one written by Gunther Frank, who is a world authority on Kombucha. You might also be interested in Alexander Solzenitzen's account of the use of Kombucha in "The Cancer Ward". In recent decades, investigation into the fungus on a scientific basis, has been carried out in the U.S.S.R. and in Germany by several researchers.

The effect of Kombucha on promoting healthy intestinal flora as well as on keeping uric acid and cholesterol soluble has made it popular in intestinal diseases, gout and cardiovascular disease. It is said to have an enhancing effect on the glands and metabolism in general.

Kombucha contains glucuronic acid which plays a significant metabolic role in the removal of metabolic waste, toxins, chemicals and drugs. as well as the vitally important regulation of lactic acid metabolism. In its conjugated form, it is part of many important biochemicals such as heparin, chondroitin-sulphuric acid, mucoitin-sulphuric acid and hyaluronic acid. These substances play a major role in the building and maintenance of cartilage, the stomach lining and the fluid of the eye, to mention just a few of their innumerable functions. Physicians who favor natural methods of prevention and healing use the substances in the treatment of eye and connective tissue diseases including arthritis and thrombophlebitis.

L-lactic acid, another component of Kombucha, has been cited in scientific literature as usually being significantly absent in the connective tissue of **cancer** patients and its presence in large amounts is said to inhibit the development of cancer. A deficiency of this acid leads to fermentation in the metabolic processing of sugar (recall the discussion of Dr. Otto Warburg's Nobel Prize-winning discovery of cancer cell metabolism elsewhere in this book), as well as failure in cell respiration and death. L-lactic acid lowers blood pH toward the acid range and thus creates an environment opposite to the alkaline pH seen in cancer pattients.

Kombucha cultures can be purchased with complete instructions on how to propagate it in the home indefinitely and with comparative ease. It grows fairly rapidly and produces enough "offspring" to supply all your neighbors in short order.

****

157

MAITAKE MUSHROOM

In Japan, the **Maitaki mushroom** (Grifola frondosa) has been found to be effective in inhibiting the growth of tumors. Its effect occurs by the stimulation of the immune system (natural killer cells, interleukin-1 and cytotoxic T-cells).

As an interesting addition to the on-going expose of the great AIDS-AZT fraud, documents of the National Cancer Institute in 1991 revealed that **Maitake mushrooms** were as effective in inhibiting the growth of the so-called HIV virus equally as well as the toxic killer drug AZT. Incredibly, **the National Cancer Institute converted the natural Maitaki extract into a sulphate and thus rendered it toxic.** AZT continues to make billions for the Wellcome Company, while committing mass murder. Other mushroom products have been obstructed by the FDA in spite of the fact that they have proved effective against cancer in other parts of the world. PSK, widely used throughout the world, has been blocked by the FDA. (You are better off with the Maitake mushroom itself, so bon appetit!)

I. Hishida, et al. Antitumor activity exhibited by orally administered extract from the fruit body of Grifola frondosa **(Maitake).** (Chem Pharm Bull (Tokyo) 1988.)

K. Adachi, et al. Potentiation of host-mediated antitumor activity in mice by beta-glucan obtained from Grifola frondosa **(Maitake).** Chem Pharm Bull (Tokyo) 1987. N. Ohno, et al. Two different confirmations of antitumor glucans obtained from Grifola frondosa. (Chem Pharm Bull (Tokyo) 1986.)

References about isolating "active ingredients" (But remember, the mushrooms work and are cheaper):

Y. Kabir, et al. Effect of **Shiitake** (Lentinus edodes) and **Maitake** (Grifola frondosa) mushrooms on blood pressure and plasma lipids of spontaneously hypertensive rats. (J Nutr Sci Vitaminol (Tokyo) 1987.)

C. Henderson, **Illudin S** may have specific cytotoxicity (mushroom derivative drug). (NCI Cancer Weekly 1990.)

T. Ikekawa, et al. Studies on antitumor polysaccharides of **Flammulina velutipes** (Curt. ex Fr.) Sing.II. The structure of EA3 and further purification of EA5. (J. Pharmacobiodyn. 1982)

M.J. Kelner, et al., Pre-clinical evaluation of **illudins** as anticancer agents. (Cancer Res. 1987.)

M.J. Kelner, et al., Pre-clinical evaluation of **illudins** as anticancer agents: basis for selective cytotoxicity. (J Natl Cancer Inst. 1990.)

K. Kino. et al. Isolation and characterization of a new immunomodulatory protein, ling zhi-8 (LZ-8), from Ganorma m. (J.Biol. Chem. 1989.)

H. Maruyama, et al. **Antitumor** activity of Sarcodon aspratus (Berk.) S. Ito and Ganoderma lucidum (Fr.) Karst. J. (Pharmacobiodyn. 1989.)

H. Nishino, et al. Studies on interrelation of structure and **antitumor** effects of polysaccharides: antitumor action of periodate-modified, branched (1-3)-beta-D-glucan of Auricularia auricula-judae, and other polysaccharides containing (1-3)-glycosidic linkages. (Carbohydr. Res. 1981.)

I. Nono, et al. Modification of **immunostimulating** activities of grifolan by the treatment with (1-3)-beta-D-gluconase. (J. Pharmacobiodyn. 1989.)

F. al Obeidi, et al. Synthesis and actions of a melanotropin conjugate, Ac-(Nle4, Glu (gamma-4'-hydroxyanilide) 5, D-Phe7) alpha-MSH4-10-NH2, on melanocytes and **melanoma** cells in vitro. (J. Pharm Sci. 1990.)

K. Otagiri, et al., Intensification of **antitumor-immunity** by protein bound polysaccharide, EA6, derived from Flammulina velutipes (Curt. ex Fr.) Sing. combined with murine leukemia L1210 vaccine in animal experiments, (J Pharmacobiodyn. 1983.)

T. Sasaki, et al. Antitumor polysaccharides from some polyporaceae Ganoderma applantum (Pers.) Pat and Phellinus linteus (Berk. et Curt) Aoshima. (Chem Pharm Bull (Tokyo). 1971.)

I. Suzuki, et al. **Antitumor** and immunomodulating activities of a beta-glucan obtained from liquid-cultured Grifola frondosa. (Chem Pharm Bull (Tokyo). 1989.)

M. Takehara, et al. Antiviral activity of virus-like particles from Lentinus edodes (Shiitake). (Brief report. Arch Virol. 1979.)

M. Takerhara, et al. **Antitumor** effect of virus-like particles from Lentinus edodes (Shiitake) on **Ehrlich ascites carcinoma** in mice. (Arch Virol. 1981.)

159

T. Takeyama, et al. Host-mediated **antitumor** effect of grifolan NMF-5N, a polysaccharide obtained from Grifola frondosa. (J. Pharmacobiodyn. 1987.)

****

REISHI MUSHROOM

A fungus, the Reishi mushroom, has received increased attention because of recent studies in the far east 190
indicating **immuno-potentiation** in mice. China, Japan and Korean scientists have discovered evidence of adaptogenic action, anti-allergenic properties, cholesterol reduction action and anti-tumor activity.

The **Reishi mushroom** inhibits tumor growth (H. Maruyama in the journal of Pharmacobiodynamics, 1989). The various chemical components of mushrooms, i.e. lectins, polysaccharides, glucans and lentinan have yielded extracts in drugs that are proving to be effective as **anti-cancer** and anti-infectious agents. Of course, this is all well and good, but I think it makes a lot more sense to make a wide variety of mushrooms, a part of your diet. Besides, there are no "side effects".

****

SHIITAKE MUSHROOM

The **Shiitake mushroom** of China was popular as medicinal during the Ming dynasty of China during the 14th century. It has been estimated that fifty varieties of mushroom have **anti-carcinogenic** effects. H. Nanba, et al. Antitumor action of shiitake (Lentinus edodes) fruit bodies orally administered to mice. Chem Pharm Bull (Tokyo) 1987.

****

TEAS

PAU D'ARCO

Almost every health food store has Pau d'arco tea on their shelves. It has long been a folk remedy in the treatment of **cancer**. It is also commonly known as Taheebo, Lapacho and Iperoxo. It has been used for many diseases, such as bronchitis, asthma, diabetes, malaria and tuberculosis. In recent years, evidence is emerging that it may be helpful in **breast cancer, sarcomas, carcinomas and leukemias**. However, very little is available in the scientific literature (J. B. Block, Cancer Chemotherapy, 1974).

DON'T FORGET GREEN TEA! - Page 75

****

SEAWEED

The Japanese have eaten sea vegetation for centuries, so it is not unusual that all scientific investigation in this area is Japanese. One plant called by the Japanese, **"Viva Natural"**, is an immune stimulant and has been found to be effective in treating **leukemia** and **lung cancer** (E. Furusawa, Oncology, 1978 and B. Sokoloff, Oncology, 1989). It has also been found to be anti-viral and has been used in combination with the chemotherapy and an extract from the narcissus plant called PTZ.

There have been indications that vegetables from the sea play a role in protecting women from **breast cancer**, primarily through stimulation of the immune system, as well as standard nutritional effects (J. Teas, Medical Hypotheses, 1981).

Dr. Teas also examined **Laminaria**, a high fiber plant which also seemed to play a roll in the prevention of **breast cancer** (Nutr. Cancer 1983 and Cancer Res. 1984).

I. Yamamoto, in the Journal of Experimental Medicine, 1984, in Japan, investigated an extract from brown sea algae which proved to be effective against leukemia.

As a food, sea vegetables are extremely nutritious and, unless

161

eaten in extremely large amounts, is safe like any other food.

****

SPICES

Yellow Ginger (Turmeric) was reported by R. Kuttan to exhibit anti-cancer activity (Cancer Lett. 1985). He also wrote of its topical use in cancer therapy, in Tumori. 1987. N.T. Huang experimented with **skin tumors** in mice and found that it had an inhibition rate of 98% (Cancer Research, 1988). D.K. Shalini demonstrated that turmeric provided **DNA protection** from oxidative damage by carcinogens. Excessive use can be toxic (L. A. Donatis, Biochemical Pharmacology, 1990).

Other spices which exhibit **anti-cancer effects** are:

**SESAME ASAFOETIDA DRUMSTICK LEAVES
PONNAKANNI BASIL POPPY SEEDS
CINNAMON MANATHAKKALI CUMIN SEEDS
TUMERIC GARLIC KANDATHIPILI LEAVES**

(M. Kanari, Chem.Pharm. Bull 1989, K. Aruna, Indian Journal of Experimental Biology 1990).

AND DON'T FORGET ...

The following aforementioned products can be mixed with recipes, used for flavoring and put in fruit drinks. Be inventive!

ALGAE	**SPIRULINA**
AMINO ACIDS	**CHLORELLA**
HERBAL TEAS	**AMYGDALIN**
LINSEED OIL	**BEE POLLEN**
ALOE	**ALMOND OIL**
HERBS	**SOY PRODUCTS**
VITAMIN C	

For example; amino acids are sold as flavorings for all kinds of dishes; vitamin C can be used for sour flavoring (but don't heat it); soy is used instead of salt; amygdalin for bitterness (careful on the amount) and aloe can be purchased as a juice.

Chapter 13

Other Significant Therapies

ANTINEOPLASTONS (BURZINSKI)

Stanislaw R. Burzinski, MD, Phd., a high controversial but respected physician, working in Houston, Texas, has succeeded in publishing many articles about substances he calls antineoplastons. These substances are normally found in blood and urine but appear to be lacking in patients with cancer. He has isolated several of them, and when used therapeutically they shrink a variety of cancers. His papers have appeared in esoteric journals, which are rarely read by practising physicians. Consequently, the average physician has virtually no knowledge of Dr. Burzinski's work and the successes he has had.

His work has been confirmed by L. B. Hendry and T. G. Muldoon (J Steroid Biochem. 1988), N. Eriguchi (J Japan Soc Cancer Ther. 1988), K. Hashimoto, et al., (J. Japan Soc Cancer Ther. 1990) and D.Samid, a researcher at the Uniformed Services University of Health Sciences in Maryland (Department of Defense). The treatment is virtually devoid of side effects and should be combined with other treatments presented in this book, depending upon the type of tumor. I have met Dr. Burzinski and have heard him lecture. He is brilliant, sincere and dedicated.

****

CANCELL

The story of cancell is a remarkable one. Its method of manufacture and its composition remains a secret. Until recently cancell could be gotten free by any one. I understand the FDA has stopped the production and distribution. It was developed by Jim Sheridan in the 1930's, who was a chemist with the Dow Chemical Company. Sheridan claims that the testing of Cancell has been blocked by the American Cancer Society in 1953 and in 1982 and again in 1986 by the Food and Drug Administration (FDA - USA). Cancell has been given free all these years to cancer patients. I have heard a fair number of success stories in my travels. Ed Sopcak a Michigan business-man, has been making and distributing it free. I read that in early 1993 the FDA got the courts to stop him. So what's new? Cancell is a natural catechol that inhibits cell respiration and forces the cancer cell into completely primitive metabolism, in which state it can be disposed of by the body's normal defenses. Results take approximately a month and vitamin C and E should not be taken in large amounts with it.

****

CARNIVORA

An extract of the Venus Fly Trap (Dionea muscipula), Carnivora digest protein. It was discovered by Dr. Helmut Keller (M.D.). There is a fair amount of scientific literature on plumbagin, a non-toxic constituent if the extract.

In India, M. Krishnaswamy, K.K. Purushothaman, and B. Chandrasekaran have published studies in the Journal of Biochemical Biophysics (India) in 1980 and 1982 demonstrating **anticancer** activity of plumbagin. Other studies have shown plumbagin to be effective in skin healing (from Plumbago scandens) and was published in 1974 by A.M. Melo (Rev Inst Antibiot).

In Russia it is used a food preservative and is harmless (V.G. Ingre. 1978). The substance must be purified properly and can be taken by mouth, inhaled or injected. The dose varies according to administration. Dr. Keller is now located in Bad

Steben, Germany. For those who plan to travel to Germany to see Dr. Keller I have a thought to consider: You can't bake a cake with flour alone. Let Carnivora be only a part of your therapy.

****

COLON CLEANSING

The waste matter that accumulates in the large bowel can commonly collect over extremely long periods of time. It may be difficult to believe, but it can retain sticky, rubbery black matter that has been there for as much as 20 - 30 years. These deposits of waste can extend to the point where they can coat the entire large and even small intestine. The transit of time of a very long intestinal tract has become more of a problem since humans started eating refined foods with less fiber. This poisonous fecal material causes mucus to drain out of the bowel. It prevents the cells from performing their normal detoxifying and filtering functions. It is obvious why so many health authorities believe that putrefaction, fermentation and incrustation of the lower bowel can have an impact on every ailment known to man and it coincides directly with the finding that the lack of adequate fiber in the diet, which increases its transit time, is related to the occurrence of **colon cancer**. The lower bowel contains high concentrations of disease-producing bacteria, toxins, waste ferments and chemicals that seep into the blood stream and lymphatic system and are transported to every part of the body. Because of the crustation it creates, large amounts of mucus are formed and the absorption of nutrients is further hindered. The body becomes auto-intoxicated because toxic waste is absorbed back into the body. Symptoms associated with self-poisoning are:

1. Halitosis

2. Body Odor

3. Headaches

4. Skin eruptions such as Acne, rashes, boils, etc.

5. Mood swings including anxiety, irritation, depression.

6. Constipation, hard stools, diarrhea (what appears to be rapid transit of waste matter and fluids through the bowel, is actually caused by the contractions of the bowel trying to compensate for the improper functioning caused by the old waste and crustations.

ALIMENTARY (DIGESTIVE TRACT) TOXEMIA

The Royal Society of Medicine in England, held a conference in which the subject of Alimentary Toxemia was discussed. One or more of thirty-six poisons and toxins were mentioned. Actual experience, not theoretical guessing, was the basis for the list of conditions that could result from this condition. They are:

EYES
Dullness of the eyes, heaviness of the eyes, inflammation of the lens and optic nerve, iritis, cataracts, iridocyclitis sclerotitis, sclerokeratitis, hardening of the lens, retinal hemorrhage.

SKIN
Wrinkling, loss of elasticity, dermatitis, acne, boils, eczema, herpes, lupus, pigmentations, seborrhea, psoriasis, dark circles under the eyes.

MUSCLES AND JOINTS
Acute and chronic arthritis, muscular rheumatism and pain, abdominal muscle weakness (causing greater constipation), bone deformities, tubercular and rheumatoid arthritis, spinal curvature, pes planus (flat feet).

CARDIOVASCULAR DISEASE
Arteriosclerosis, hypertension (high blood pressure), low blood pressure, myocarditis, endocarditis, heart enlargement, dilation of the aorta, peripheral vascular disease.

DIGESTIVE TRACT

Tooth decay, mouth ulcers, gingival (gums) infection, pharyngeal (throat) ulcers, pyloric spasm and obstruction, dilation, distention, inflammation, ulceration and **cancer of the stomach,** gallstones and **cancer of the gall bladder,** degeneration, inflammation, cirrhosis and **cancer of the liver,** inflammation and **cancer of the pancreas,** enlargement of the spleen, adhesions and obstruction (kinking) of the small intestine.

GENITO-URINARY TRACT

Mastitis, fibrosis and **cancer of the breast,** bladder and kidney infections, displacements of the kidney and uterus, frequent urination, uterine disease.

MISCELLANEOUS

Growth retardation in children, premature senility, lowered resistance to infection **(immune deficiency),** degeneration of the kidneys, liver and spleen and **various tumors.**

- believe it or not!

TECHNIQUES

Professional Colonics - Though somewhat expensive, this help is strongly advised for at least the first couple of cleansings. It can be difficult to dislodge waste material that has impacted in the furrows of the bowel interior.

Home Cleansing - Standard enema equipment which can be purchased anywhere will suffice. It is recommended that a flow control that can be reduced to where a quart or liter of solution will take fifteen minutes be used. This permits time for the fluid to work its way throughout the colon and does not cause discomfort. The enema should be taken in a kneeling position with the shoulders lowered to the bed or the floor (knee-chest position). Bottled water is advised, very warm but not hot. Add 2 to 6 tablespoons of hydrogen peroxide 3%. I prefer freshly ozonated water - ozonated during administration.

Laxatives - Herbal preparations are preferred. An excellent preparation consists of:

Butternut Bark of Root (White Walnut-Juglans cinerea)
Cascara Sagrada Bark (Rhamnus purshiana)
Rhubarb Root (Rheum palmatum) Ginger Root (Zingiber officinale)
Licorice Root (Glycyrrhiz glabra)
Irish Moss (Chondrus crispus)
Cayenne (Capsicum annuum)

Preparation: approximately 4000 mg, per capsule.

Use: This preparation is effective yet mild enough for children. It should be taken with a light meal.

Dose:

age 5-7,	1 capsule twice daily.
age 8-12,	2 capsule three times daily.
age 13-19,	2 capsules three to four times daily.
age 20-55,	2 to 3 capsules every four hours.
age 56 & up,	1 to 2 capsules twice daily.

****

GERSON THERAPY

Dr. Max Gerson takes his place of honor in the history of modern medicine because he has, like many other notable physicians, been attacked by the American Medical Association. It will be recorded one day, that if you wish to find a list of scientists who have truly contributed most to the development of effective non-toxic therapies, you simply have to look at a list of the victims of AMA treachery and viciousness. (fostered by the pharmaceutical industry and aided and abetted by our unfaitful servants at the FDA). Max Gerson's "crime" was that he advocated the use of coffee enemas which, surprisingly, has a scientific rationale and is based on research done in Germany in the 1920's. It could even be found in the Merck Manual during its first twenty years of publication. The American Medical Association, in its usual attitude of arrogance and ignorance, claimed that there was no scientific evidence that the "modification with a dietary intake of food or other nutritional essentials of any specific use in the control of cancer". Today, the AMA still lobbies the United States Congress as the outstanding authority on what is good for the health of the American public.

Gerson's program consisted of a diet high in organic fruits, vegetables and grains and low in animal proteins and fat. He supplemented the diet with potassium and iodine and advocated the use of raw liver juice.

Gerson was particularly ridiculed by advocating the use of **coffee enemas**. The actions of this therapy are actually multiple. The caffeine in the coffee is carried directly to the portal vein from the rectum where it stimulates activity by the liver which is the major detoxificating organ in the body.

L. K. Lamb, in the Journal of Medical Chemistry, 1987, commented on the **anti-cancer** agents present in coffee.

The use of enemas for cleansing the bowl go back to pre-Biblical times. The only comments that I have seen of a pseudo-scientific nature, appeared in a journal I read many years ago, where the author derided their use by stating that they would draw needed minerals out of the body. This is, of course, absolute nonsense and cannot be substantiated by any scientific evidence. Considering the number of "side effects" of most laxatives and the amount taken by individuals yearly, it is laxatives that should be abandoned and enemas be reinstituted as a recommended medical therapy.

Gerson stressed the harmfulness of sodium in the diet and his position has been confirmed by B. Jansson, whose articles in the past ten years stressed the relationship of the sodium potassium ratio and the occurrence of cancer. Jansson recommends the dietary ratio for potassium to sodium one-to-one. This is not difficult to accomplish if we eliminate the salt shaker from the table and commercially prepared foods.

I do not feel that the Gerson therapy is sufficient by itself as an answer to the treatment of cancer. However, the basic principles of nutrition which Gerson expounded, are certainly an essential guideline for diet and are undoubtedly effective in prevention as well as treatment. I would strongly advise the addition of the Budwig formula.

****

GLANDULARS

Although, in the section under cell-therapy, I discussed, "glandulars", I think it important to relate that extracts, both liquid and powder, from edible animals, can provide beneficial therapeutic effects. In particular, organs dealing with the immune defenses, are good choices to take, either in tablet form, or eaten as part of a meal. Of course, the problem today is to find thymus, liver, spleen or other organs that have not been contaminated by feeds or pastures that have been laced with poisonous fertilizers and pesticides. For individuals that cannot afford cell-therapy, I strongly advise the use of simple glandulars as making a great deal of sense and backed by many scientific articles, too great to even think of listing completely.

Hormones are often a combination of substances, or "factors". The thyroid, thymus and spleen have various components which have been synthesized, so that certain fractions can be used for different disease processes (L. Denes, Cancer Immunol Immunother. 1990). The problem with most of the information we are given, is that studies of commercially produced factors, are financially attractive, but rarely do they ever compare them with the simple, inexpensive whole glandular, naturally occurring organ.

Extracts from the thymus gland contain factors that are labelled, Thymosin, Thymopoietin and Thymopentin, can individually be shown to cause or prevent specific effects. For example, G. L. Cartia, in 1990, demonstrated that Thymopentin protected women with breast cancer from the destructive effects of chemotherapy.

Thymosin seemed to be most helpful in infectious problems and, in one study, against the dissemination of malignant melanoma (I.F. Labunets, 1989).

****

HOXSEY THERAPY

In the middle part of this century, Harry Hoxsey stirred up more controversy than any other individual in the area of alternative therapies for cancer. His cause was championed in the United States Congress by Senators and Congressmen. The story has been related that Hoxsey had a running battle with the notoriously discredited Morris Fishbein of the American Medical Association and editor of their journal. The Office of Technology Assessment, a branch of the United States Congress, in 1990, many years after Hoxsey's death, admitted that Hoxsey's formula contained many substances that had proven therapeutic activity. The United States government and the FDA viciously attacked Hoxsey and spent many hundreds of thousands of dollars in trying to discredit and destroy Hoxsey. It is no different than the same tactics they use today, at even greater expense, to destroy therapies known to be effective and backed by scientific evidence. Many fine researchers and physicians have lost everything in trying to battle these all too obvious representatives of the Pharmaceutical industry.

Hoxsey's formula contained **burdock** which has been confirmed by the World Health Organization to have an anti-viral effect.

K. Morita, et al., in Mutation Research, 1984, discovered that burdock could reduce the harmful effects of substances that caused mutations.

Another ingredient of the formula is **poke root** which has been used medically as an anti-parasitic and anti-rheumatic. (The Merck Index).

M. P. Bodger in Immunology 1979, demonstrated that pokeweed stimulated the **immune system**. R. A. Owens in Virology, 1973, wrote of its viricidal ability. T. Y. Bashim demonstrated that it could stimulate the thymus and the production of interleukin.

J. P. Jang, in a Chinese journal in 1990, found it to be better than BCG (tuberculosis vaccine) in its **anti-cancer** activity.

Still another ingredient, **barberry**, was shown by A. Hoshi to have **anti-cancer**, anti-bacterial and anti-malarial activity.

S.M. Kupchan wrote of the **anti-leukemic** effect of buckthorn in mice. Buckthorn is still another ingredient in the Hoxsey formula.

Prickly ash bark and **stillingia**, two other ingredients, have not shown anti-cancer activity but do show cathartic, anti-inflammatory and pain ameliorating effects. (M.A. Oriowo, Planta Med. 1982 and G. X. Hong, 1983).

F. E. Mohs reported in JAMA, 1948, a chemosurgical treatment for **cancer of the skin**. Hoxsey had created a salve, remarkably similar, that contained zinc chloride, antimony trisulfide and bloodroot. The Office of Technology Assessment reported that Mohs claimed a "99% cure rate for all primary **basal cell carcinomas**". This therapy is still being ignored while expensive mutilating surgery still holds reign.

****

HYDRAZINE SULPHATE

Dr. Joseph Gold, in the 1970's, reported that hydrazine sulphate inhibited the growth of cancers in rats, including **melanoma, lymphoma and leukemia** (Oncology, 1971 and 1973).

Based on Otto Warburg's Nobel Prize-winning discovery, that anaerobic glycolysis or the fermentation process was the means by which cancer thrived, Gold postulated that depriving cancer cells of glucose could stop tumor growth. In an article in Oncology, 1975, Gold's study involving patients with terminal cancer, demonstrated marked improvements in all cancer-related parameters, i.e. stabilization of weight, increased energy, appetite and daily activities and decrease in pain. A constant important observance throughout all the studies, was maintenance or increase in weight. This finding was confirmed by studies done at UCLA and reported by Chlebowski, in Cancer Research, 1984.

J.A. Tayek reported in Lancet, the benefits to **lung cancer** patients, who were severely malnourished.

V. Filov, in a large Leningrad study, involving over seven hundred patients with many different types of cancer, not only showed better maintenance of weight, but a regression of tumor in 10%. The Russian study indicated that the best results were achieved in patients with **breast cancer, Hodgkin's Disease, neuroblastoma, laryngeal cancer and desmosarcoma.**

Can you imagine that the National Cancer Institute has belittled and discouraged the use of hydrazine sulfate, despite its non-toxicity and obvious benefits. The only reason that I can think of, that they have taken this position, is because hydazine sulfate is inexpensive and cannot be patented.

****

IMMUNO-AUGMENTATIVE THERAPY (IAT)

The Story of IAT is another saga of controversy, conflict and confusion. Lawrence Burton Ph.D. has been involved in scientific disputes since the 1950's, when he and his co-workers claimed to have discovered a "Tumor Induction Factor". His findings appeared in Cancer Research, 1956 and Science in 1956 and 1962.

In the early 1960's, he published papers on cancer-inhibiting substances which appeared in the Proceedings of the American Association for Cancer Research and The New York Academy of Sciences.

IAT consists of administering antitumor antibodies centrifuged from the blood. The Burton Clinic which is located Freeport in the Bahamas, has been opened and closed on several occasions under pressure from U.S. authorities. In 1986, there was a scare because of alleged HIV contamination. At the time there were doubts as to the validity of the charges and with the unfolding of the "AIDS" fraud, I am sure the attack was unjustified. The closest personal knowledge I have of Burton's therapy was from an individual in Florida who had improved remarkably and from conversations with a doctor in Mexico who had worked at a franchised satellite clinic in Tijuana. The Mexican clinic was run originally by a cancer survivor and was last under the direction of his son who according to this physician was **not** following Burton's protocol. My experience in Tijuana leads me to believe the physician. I would trust the doctors there, but not the entrepreneurs. Those individuals contemplating a trip to Tijuana are advised to follow my recommendations in the Resource section of this book.

****

KOCH THERAPY

In the first decades of the twentieth century, Dr. Robert Koch developed a protocol for the treatment of cancer using Glyoxilic acid. Although its use was stopped by the FDA in the United States in the 1940's, the treatment can be obtained in Europe and some Latin American countries, including Mexico. The Koch therapy is based on the oxidative process. The effect of oxygen on the biochemistry of the cell promotes the destruction of pathogens and restores the cell to its normal state. By using compounds judicially and in safe amounts, Koch worked out a program utilizing minute amounts (2 millimicrograms) of **SSR (Synthetic Survival Reagent, a carbonyl compound) and benzoquinone to facilitate the oxidation process.** Some clinics in Mexico are using the Koch therapy adjunctively with Laetrile.

Koch stressed a diet similar to the diet that Dr. Johanna Budwig advocates, and which is utilized by most alternative cancer clinics with varying degrees of strictness. Koch was adamant in denouncing the use of aspirin and any other coal tar derivatives as they hinder the oxygen carrying capacity of the blood. He advocated vitamin A in the form of fish oils and cautioned against the use of Beta-carotine in large amounts in cancer patients, as they are not able to oxidize it to create vitamin A (remember: Beta-carotene is useful as a preventative and vitamin A for treatment).. He also advocated colonics and the ingestion of raw vegetables (or lightly cooked) to keep the bowels moving. Selenium is necessary in the diet, but Koch pointed out that there was danger of toxicity if judicious use was ignored. He recommended lactobacillus be added to the diet and that food be chewed well in order that enzymatic action can take place.

It is claimed that the Koch treatment is effective in a wide range of diseases including tuberculosis, infections in general, cardiovascular disease, allergy, psoriasis etc. Considering the biochemistry involved, it may very well be so.

****

THE LIVINGSTON THERAPY

Because allopathic medicine is so bogged down and blinded by the hypotheses that organisms cause everything (germ theory), it is surprising that the work of Virginia Livingston wasn't taken more seriously. She believed that the microbe she observed under the microscope and which she named Progenitor cryptocides, was the cause of cancer. This tiny organism has been seen and written about by hundreds of investigators. Respected scientists agree with Livingston's hypothesis. I suspect that Naessen's Somatides are one and the same (See 714-X). Both describe their organism as changing its shape and behavior. My guess is that there is validity to both theoretical roles ascribed to them in that these changes are directed by the many known carcinogens in our environment. They could play a role in the conversion of the cellular genetic material to a less differentiated state.

Another interesting claim, not supported by scientific literature, was made by Dr. Livingston, that **abscisic acid,** a plant hormone, was nature's strongest weapon against cancer.

Livingston's treatment was stopped by the State of California authorities in 1990, just before she died. Her treatment consisted of making a patient-specific vaccine of P. cryptocides (orally and subcutaneously); the administration of gamma globulin; BCG and other bacterial vaccines and direct blood transfusions. She used intravenous vitamin support, and strongly advocated a vegetarian diet. Her greatest objections involved **poultry, sugar, refined flour, processed foods, smoking and alcohol.**

****

MACROBIOTICS

The macrobiotic diet is based upon the traditional Japanese diet. It has been popularized by Michio Kushi. Kushi linked the cause of cancer directly with diet and lifestyle. The macrobiotic diet is primarily whole grains and vegetables, to which small amounts of seaweed, fish and fruit have been added. All grains are whole grains and organically grown. Certain vegetables, such as all types of potatoes, tomatos, egg plant, avocado, zucchini, asparagus, spinach and peppers are forbidden. Proteins are provided by lentils, chickpeas and soy bean products. Coffee and tea are not allowed.

The basic approach of macrobiotics is confirmed by much of the recent scientific literature. The increase in fiber, the avoidance of red meat and the increased intake of yellow and green vegetables, the use of soy and green tea are all mentioned in scientific references (M. Masina, J Am Diet Assoc. 1991; J. Nat'l. Cancer Inst. 1991; H. Benjamin, et al., Cancer Res. 1991; J. Etas, Med. Hypotheses, 1981; D.P. Burkett, AM J Clin. Nutr., 1978).

The macrobiotic diet can result in nutritional deficiencies because it is difficult to follow and requires a wide variety of foods at each feeding. I have recommended to my patients, who followed this diet, supplementation with essential fatty acids, complete amino acid powders along with vitamins and minerals. Vitamin B12 supplementation has been found in several studies, to be a necessary supplement (G. Debry, Rev Prat. 1991; P.C. Dagnelie, Am J Clin Nutr. 1990; D.R. Mellor, et al., Am J Clin Nutr. 1991).

****

Chapter 14

Immune Stimulants

ARISTOLOCHIA ACID

In the 1960's, Professor J.R. Mose, of Austria, performed a series of experiments demonstrating that Aristolochia stimulated the production of phagocytes without a concomitant increase in the other leucocytes (white blood cells) in the blood. The phagocytes are particularly significant in that these "killer-cells" are known to attack all foreign invaders as well as cells which are abnormal to the system i.e. **cancer cells**. Prof. Mose also noted that the phagocytes were able to ingest larger amounts of foreign material than usual. This is a strong indication of immune response.

Experiments have shown that Aristolochia Acid inhibited growth of artificially induced tumors in laboratory animals. It has also been used on a long lasting basis as a preventative measure in cancer.

In infections, Aristolochia is utilized as a **Eubiotic**, in that it stimulates the body's own defenses (reticulo-endothelial system) for a therapeutic response. This is in contrast to antibiotics which kill or stunt the growth of bacteria, but at the same time have an immune suppressive effect.

Dr. Byron W. Goldberg, in the United States, tested **KC2** (aristolochia) on patients with acute leukemia, chronic aleuke-mic leukemia (granulytic series) and chronic lymphocytic leukemia. Although no significant changes were observed in the blood tests, the patients improved clinically and in quality of life. Notably, the patients exhibited resistence to infections and

177

their ability to "throw off colds". As a result, he tested KC2 (1-2 tablets every two hours while awake) on patients with "colds" and noted rapid improvement with normalization of all symptoms and body function.

In instances where antibiotics are truly indicated, Aristolochia Acid can be used instead of, or in conjunction with anti-microbial agents. It is indicated particularly in patients who are in a weakened state as a result of radiation, chemotherapy or long-term antibiotic or steroid (cortisone) therapy. It improves secondary wound healing (post-surgery).

In Europe it is known also as KC2 and can be obtained as an enteric coated tablet, liquid (for children) or ointment. When used as directed, there are no known risks or incapatibilities. The only known unwanted direct effect is a rare instance of nausea, vomiting, diarrhea or palpitations. These symptoms cease when the preparation is discontinued.

****

BESTATIN

This immune stimulant was isolated from Streptomyces olvoreticuli. It is an amino acid compound which works on cell membranes by effecting enzyme action. **Its anti-cancer effect** is obtained through the stimulation of T-cells, macrophages and certain bone marrow cells.

It has been used in **melanoma and lung cancer** (I. Saiki, Japanese Journal of Cancer Research, 1989), and in combination with other chemotherapies in **leukemia** (S. Tsukagoshi, 1987).

If the immune system has been destroyed by X-ray or other forms of radiation, Bestatin will not be effective (K. Shibuya, et al., 1987).

Although its **effectiveness** has been mainly in **blood cancers** and other blood diseases, promise is evident in **head, neck, esophageal, stomach, lung and bladder cancers**, as well as **malignant melanoma** (K. Ota, Biomed Pharmacother. 1991).

It has been used in conjunction with Levamisole, another immune stimulator, in laboratory mice, with good effect (R.M. Bruley, Immunology, 1979).

Bestatin prolongs the effect of the body's own pain killers and has been shown by G. Mathe to inhibit the breakdown of enkephalin, the body's own rapid pain-killer. (Biomed Pharmacother. 1991).

In a study done by H. Blongren and reported in Acta Oncol. 1990, it was demonstrated that Bestatin was as effective as radiation therapy, in the treatment of bladder cancer.

****

COLEY'S TOXINS

The use of bacterial toxins to stimulate the immune system, and thus provide a possible therapy for cancer, was discovered a century ago by William B. Coley, M.D. The toxins which bear his name, cause a classical toxic response which causes temperature to rise and chills, palpitations and headaches to occur. These are the natural responses of the immune system. Therapy was **effective in bone tumors (giant cell), malignant melanoma, ovarian cancer and Hodgkin's Disease.**

Dr. Frances Havas of Temple University School of Medicine, has carried on a thirty year study, confirming the usefulness of Coley's Toxins and has published many articles which have appeared in Cancer Research and other journals, spanning the years from 1958 until the present. Dr. Havas has made an observation which alternative physicians have known for decades. If patients are given antibiotics unnecessarily, the immune system cannot respond as well to stimulation.

A. R. Kean and R W. Frelick have expressed the opinion that naturally occurring fevers from infection, are as effective as the use of immune stimulants (J. Biol Res Mod. 1990). This should make you think twice about taking drugs to suppress fever.

When Coley's Toxins are used in conjunction with conventional surgery, radiation and chemotherapy, survival was increased (Y. T. Zhao, Med Oncol & Tumor Pharmacother.1991).

****

GOSSYPOL

Gossypol has been used in China, as a male oral contraceptive. It is a pigment obtained from cotton seed.

Its use in **reproductive cancers,** in both men and women, has been confirmed by studies done by V. Band, et al., and reported in Gynecological Oncology, 1989.

Leukemia and **pancreatic cancer** in mice were affected significantly by gossypol. Human breast cancer seemed to be affected also (M. Thomas, Anti-Cancer Research, 1991, S. K. Majundar, et al., 1991).

Scientists at the National Institute of Health, reported a case of **adrenal cortex cancer**, in which gossypol effected a marked decrease in **lung and liver metastases.**

****

INOSINE

The inosine molecule, which is a major chemical in the structure of DNA, is found in meat and beets. Inosine and **thymodine,** another DNA molecule, have been used with methotrexate, a chemotherapeutic antimetabolite, allowing larger doses of that agent to be administered, with less toxicity. As usual, they combine these natural substances with other chemicals to create a patentable drug, results in toxicity (J. Kaufman and A. Mittelman, Cancer Chemother Rep. 1975).

A.J. Glasky and J. Gordon, in 1986, found that a commercial preparation of inosine could protect patients from the immune defects caused by cancer chemotherapy and radiation.

It has also been found to boost survival in laboratory animals injected with cancer cells, when combined with Interferon (I. Cerutti, et al., Int J Immunopharmacol. 1979).

****

KRESTIN

A Japanese product, Krestin is extracted from common mushrooms, has been in use since 1973. **It is the most widely** used drug for cancer in the world. In the United States, however, the FDA is still "protecting" the public from the safety of this natural drug.

When used in conjunction with cancer chemotherapy, it prolongs survival by protecting the immune system (T. Fujii, et al., Oncology, 1989; and S. Tsukgoshi, Cancer Treat Rev. 1984).

It has been used effectively in combination therapy against **leukemia** (T. Nagao, et al., 1981).

T. Ando, et al., has established that Krestin improves resistence to infection, which is always a threat in cancer.

In **stomach cancer**, Krestin has been administered successfully, along with 5-FU. (H. Nakazato, et al., 1989).

****

LENTINAN

This extract from the **Shiitake mushroom** has been in use for almost thirty years. It has been successfully employed against a variety of tumors in laboratory animals. Lentanin has been used, like so many immune modulators, to protect against the "side effects" of chemotherapeutic agents. This combination has been found effective in **stomach, colorectal** and **breast cancers** (K. Okuyama, et al., Cancer, 1985 and T. Taguchi, 1983).

More importantly, it has been found effective in **preventing cancers which are caused by chemicals and viruses** (G. Chihara, et al., Int J Tissue React.1982).

In spite of the dozens of articles that have been written about the effectiveness of Lentanin in obtaining high cure rates in many cancers, and its very low toxicity, it cannot be obtained legally in the United States. However, you could always eat Shiitake mushrooms. They taste great!

****

LEVAMISOLE

Many alternative practitioners use Levamisol because it is relatively free of adverse effects. Careful monitoring of the patient is advised, however.

Studies done on Levamisole, which has long been used to de-worm animals, indicate that in combination with 5-FU, it has a significant effect in reducing the recurrence of **colon carcinoma** (C. Moertel, New England Journal of Medicine, 1990).

****

METHYLENE BLUE

This one hundred year old synthetic dye has been used in medicine, primarily as an antiseptic for the **urinary tract** and as a poison antidote.

B. T. Lai, at the Beijing Lung Tumor Research Institute, in China, in 1989, reported the effectiveness of methylene blue against three animal cancers.

It has also been demonstrated that methylene blue reaches the brain and, therefore, is potentially useful for **brain cancer**. **Phototherapy**, which is used in the treatment of **bladder** cancer, is enhanced with methylene blue (D.S. Yu, Journal of Neurology, 1990).

M.J. Kelner, in Basic Life Sciences, 1988, reported that free radical activity is inhibited by methylene blue. This medicinal is inexpensive and legal. However, because it is no longer patentable, nobody seems to be pushing it.

****

MONOCLONAL ANTIBODIES

Genetic cloning of antibodies, in which a variety of different cells are brought together, result in the creation, biologically, of cells with new characteristics that can be aimed at the destruction of cancer. The possibilities are endless. Cells can be developed that can directly invade and destroy tumors; act as messengers and carriers for drugs, toxins, etc.; produce new species for vaccines and for the production and replacement of normal cells that have been destroyed. In over twenty years, monoclonal antibodies have only been shown to have an extended effect in the treatment of **lymphoma** (R. O. Dillman, 1984).

There have been some benefits, though not impressive, demonstrated in leukemia, neuroblastoma and melanoma (R. Dillman, Rev Oncol Hematol. 1984) . It is still to early to recommend otherwise.

****

MTH-68

The use of viruses to destroy cancer, arises from observations that viral infections have caused regressions of Burkitt's lymphoma and leukemia. Laszlo K. Csatary developed the use of this phenomenon and produced a vaccine called MTH-68. In Lancet, 1971, he reported the use of the vaccine against cancer and, for fifteen years, submitted various articles to the Journal of Medicine. He has reported beneficial effects in **prostatic, bladder and breast disease.**

It is now known that viruses can stimulate the production of tumor necrosis factor and, possibly, Interferon and Interleukin. The newest form of the vaccine is called MTH-68/N, and it is now approaching its final stage of testing. Preliminary reports are very encouraging. Parallel work with a **mumps vaccine has also obtained excellent results in thyroid, breast, uterus, rectal and skin cancers** (Y. Okuno, et al., 1977/1978 and T. Asada, Cancer, 1974).

****

MUROCTASIN

Muroctasin is derived from muramyl dipeptide which is obtained from the cell walls of bacteria. Although it is more potent than the natural substance, it has very few unwanted effects. It is a Japanese product and information is only available in German and Japanese literature.

Toxicity studies have been performed by Y. Ono and H. Kojima and their groups in 1988. The most common problems were a mild transient fever and local inflammation at the site of injection. The effective treatment dose of 90mg/kg was less than half the lowest lethal dose in animals - 200mg to 800mg per kg. (Y. Ono, 1988)

Investigators believe Muroctasin is an adjunct in the treatment of low white blood cell counts caused by chemotherapy (K. Furuse, A. Sakama, M. Takada, 1988). This investigation was performed on **lung cancer** patients at the Osaka Prefectural Habikino Hospital and the National Kinki Central Hospital for Chest Diseases (Osaka).

Muroctasin also potentiates antibiotics (T. Otani, 1988). It boosts immune activity by stimulating macrophages with the resultant increase in interleukin and colony stimulating factor (CSF) production (K. Akahani et al., 1990, S, Nagao et al., 1988). **It is a promising agent for individuals taking chemotherapy and who are prone to infection.**

****

SHARK CARTILAGE

It has been known for quite some time, that sharks do not develop cancer. The reason for this is not entirely clear. However, it was discovered that shark cartilage inhibited the growth of new blood vessels. Tumors produce a substance which stimulates a growth of blood vessels in order to receive a supply of blood for their own metabolism.

Dr. Carl Luer of the Mote Marine Laboratories indicates that a protein in very high concentrations in the cartilage is responsible for this biochemical phenomena. If angiogenesis or vascularization of the tumor is prevented, then the tumor is denied the nutrients necessary for its survival.

Investigation was carried out, using shark cartilage, to inhibit the vascularization of tumors. J. Falkman and H. Brem published articles in the Journal of Experimental Medicine in 1975 and in Scientific American in 1976 on this subject.

Dr. G. Atassi of the Institute Jules Bordet in Brussels, Belgium, experimentally demonstrated in 1989 that shark cartilage, administered by mouth, is effective in **inhibiting tumor growth.** The Chinese have been eating soup from shark cartilage (shark fin soup) for centuries without any evidence of adverse effects. Research for many years on laboratory animals has also failed to produce side effects. Therefore shark cartilage is obviously safe. There are many papers in the scientific literature supporting the use as a logical food supplement in individuals at high risk for cancer. Dr. Brian Durie, testing the effects of shark cartilage on tumor cells in the laboratory, found it to be highly effective in destroying certain cancer stem cells.

In another study on **melanoma** cells, Dr. Astassi found it to be significant in prolonging survival time. Dr. Ghanem Atassi experimented with human melanoma cells, injected into mice, which were then fed shark cartilage. The growth of tumors were markedly inhibited in the mice fed shark cartilage, as compared to the control group.

In the past two years, (1992-93) a large scale investigation was performed in Cuba with promising effects. Interviews on major television shows (60 MINUTES) were shown, in which Cuban and American investigators confirmed that there were beneficial results in cancer.

Investigation by Dr. Robert Langer, at the Massachusetts Institute of Technology, confirmed the effects of shark cartilage and submitted a paper to the Proceedings of the National Academy of Sciences in the United States, in 1980.

In 1983, an article appeared in the journal Science vol. 221 by Dr. Robert Langer in which he demonstrated that shark cartilage strongly inhibited the growth of new blood vessels (angiogenesis) toward **solid tumors** "thereby restricting tumor growth".

G. R. Pettit and R. H. Ode isolated two anti-cancer substances from shark cartilage (Journal of Pharmacological Sciences, 1977). There have been no reports of toxicity from the use of shark cartilage. However, my own investigations in Mexico, revealed that contamination, causing illness, can occur in situations where controls on manufacturing are not stringent. This is not meant to detract from the benefits, but to merely caution the reader to obtain it from a reliable source. The FDA in the United States, will release AZT, a drug that causes AIDS, for the treatment of AIDS, but will not condone shark cartilage, a food which is harmless, for the treatment of cancer!

Shark cartilage has shown to be effective in fortifying the immune system in a variety of inflammatory conditions, particularly arthritis. Professor Serge Orloff M.D. of the Brugmann University Hospital of Brussels, used the cartilage successfully in degenerative joint disease.

Other investigators have demonstrated its effectiveness in laboratory animals and humans. Studies on osteoarthritics at the Miami School of Medicine by Jose Orcasita M.D., in Costa Rica by Carlos Alpizar, M.D., head of the national geriatric program and V. Rejholec, M.D., of the Charles University in Czechoslovakia have all demonstrated dramatic results. Individual cases showing significant improvement involving Lyme disease, psoriasis, eczema and lupus erythematosus have been reported. Dosages are variable and range from 4 to 30 grams daily depending on the condition being treated. Rectal installation also appears to be an effective route of administration. Although it has not been demonstrated to be harmful in any situation, there should be some caution and physician supervision in individuals where angiogenesis is desirable, such as after recent heart attacks, in children and in pregnancy.

****

SOD

Superoxide Dismutase (SOD) like Vitamin E, Beta-Carotene and Vitamin C, is a free radical scavenger. Susceptibility to carcinogens of **breast cancer cells**, is lessened by the presence of SOD. A great deal of research involving SOD is going on, because of the roll of free radicals in many diseases.

A Chinese investigator, R. Dai, demonstrated that SOD levels were higher in healthy adults than in patients with cancer of the **breast, lung, digestive tract and the reproductive system.**

D. Glaves, in 1986, reported that SOD inhibited **lung cancer** cells.

R. Miesel and U. Weser demonstrated the anti-cancer effectiveness of a copper-SOD compound.

SOD compounds effectively reduce the side effects of radiation therapy, particularly with relation to fibrous scar tissue formation (F. Baillet, et al., 1986 and M. Housset, et al., 1989).

SOD has also been used in conjunction with tumor necrosis factor. The effectiveness of oral SOD is still disputed.

SPLENOPENTIN

Similar in activity to thymus hormone, splenopentin was initially designated as thymopoietin III. It is actually produced by the spleen. Human splenopentin proved to be more effective than bovine in studies on immunodeficiency states (V.A. Evseev et al. 1991, H.U. Simon, et al., Allerg Immunol., 1990).

According to Simon et al., splenopentin is well-tolerated. It appears to be beneficial in grafting of tissue bone marrow transplants and restoring antibody production (R. Eckert et al., Exp Clin Endocrinol. 1989 and 1990)

In a study by J. Greiner in 1990, it was found to be useful in the treatment of psoriasis and its arthritis.

At the San Bartolo Hospital in Vicenza a study on Hodgkin's disease patients showed that splenopentin and thymic hormone were equal in their immune stimulating response (T. Chisesi et al., J Biol Regul Homeost Agents. 1988).

****

VACCINES

BCG (ANTI-TUBERCOLOSIS VACCINE)

The vaccine for tuberculosis, known as BCG, is currently being used as therapy in various types of cancer, because it stimulates lymphocytes and macrophages to attack cancer cells.

It has been primarily used successfully in the treatment of **melanoma, bladder cancer, lung cancer** and **leukemia** (R. Verloes, British Journal of Cancer, 1981). The treatment is usually well tolerated. However, severe shock reactions (anaphyllaxis) have occurred. BCG has been used for over twenty years.

****

STAPHAGE LYSATE

The vaccine, Staphage Lysate, has been in use for over fifty years. Typically, it was attacked and surpressed by Establishment Medicine and the American Cancer Society. The claims by its originator, Robert E. Lincoln, MD., have been supported by scientific studies in the past decade (H.J. Esber, Immunopharmacology, 1985).

The vaccine stimulates the production of natural body Interferon, which has no side effects and far less expensive than the toxic, commercially available, Interferon. Laboratory studies indicate that Staphage Lysate should be considered as a means of stopping the spread and growth of **breast cancer** (A. Mathur, et al., Journal of Investigative Surgery, 1988).

****

MARUYAMA VACCINE

Professor Chisato Maruyama of the Nippon Medical School, in the 1960's, developed an extract from the bacteria that causes tuberculosis. The Japanes health authorities have stubbornly refused to allow this vaccine to be used outside of this one medical school, in spite of the fact that the Central Pharmaceutical Affairs Council has urged its release for use in amelioration of radiation side effects.

There have been reports of dramatic effects in **metastatic testicular cancer to the lung** (K. Fijita et al., Cancer Detect Prev. 1981). (It also appears to be effective in the treatment of hepatitis B.)

The Maruyama vaccine stimulates the production of Interferon and collagen (T. Kimoto, 1982 and Y. Hayashi, 1981). The studies in laboratory animals give evidence that the formation of collagen entraps the cancer tissue, which is a unique way of containing a tumor (H. Nagae, 1990).

The effects on the anti-tumor activity have been studied R.B. Pollard et al. (Anticancer Research 1990), F, Suzuki et al. (J Natl Cancer Inst.1986) and H. Sasaki et al.(Cancer Res 1990).

****

UREA

Urea is a natural substance found most abundantly in urine. It is oderless and colourless when chrystalized. The first evidence of **anti-cancer** activity was noted in 1941 by J. Thompson. These findings were confirmed in a large study, performed by E. Lowe and reported in Medical World in 1944. As expected, the cancer establishment in Britain denounced this inexpensive, non-patentable substance.

A medical school professor, at the Athens University, E. D. Danopoulos, revived interest in urea with a series of articles that appeared in the famous Lancet, and Clinical Oncology through the years 1974 - 1983. Dr. Danopoulos dealt mainly with **cancers of the eye**, of various types. His studies and reports indicated remarkably high success rates with actual cure. He presented many cases of **lip cancer** of different types with, again, an exceptionally high incidence of success.

Other investigators have found urea to be effective in treating **malignant melanomas** in hamsters (B. Ecanow, Clinical Oncology, 1977, and **cancers of the cervix and penis** (G. Gandi, et al., Journal of Surgical Oncology, 1977). Danopoulos recommends his treatment in early cancers of the liver and **metastatic lesions of the lung**. He advocates both **oral** administration and **injection** of a 40% solution.

****

Chapter 15

Other Products To Consider - Maybe!

(Not So Natural, Not So Safe)

ANTICOAGULANTS

Substances which interfere with the normal clotting mechanisms in the blood, have been used primarily in heart disease and in peripheral vascular disease. Warfarin, a common rat poison, and Coumadin, an extract from the Tonka bean, and other plants, are now being tested in the treatment of cancer. These substances seem to prevent tumor cells from sticking to cell walls, a process somewhat related to the formation of a clot. Using this principle, a series of clinical trials were set up world-wide. H. Ludwig, in 1974, stated that anticoagulants increased survival time of **cancer** patients to a varying degree.

****

WARFARIN

L. R. Zacharski achieved 100% increase in survival in **small cell carcinoma of the lung** with **warfarin**.

Warfarin, used in conjunction **with 5-FU,** was shown by J. Ogawa, in 1988, to work more effectively together.

****

HEPARIN

Heparin and enzymes such as **streptokinase**, have also been shown to have **anti-metastatic** effects (R.D. Thornes, Cancer, 1975 and E. Gorelik, Cancer Research, 1987). **Cortisone was** given in conjunction **with heparin** with an added anti-cancer metastatic effect (B. Astedt, 1977, J. Folkman, Science, 1983).

It is interesting to note that this "modern approach" is not at all new. A **Chinese traditional medicine called, Qian-Hu,** accomplished a similar result (it contains a form of coumarin). This finding was published in Carcinogenesis, in 1990, by J.T. Zelikoff.

Similar effects have been found using Mo-ehr, the Chinese black tree fungus and the venom of certain snakes (K. A. Knudsen, Exp Cell Res. 1988, J. George and S. Shattil, The New England Journal of Medicine, 1991).

****

NAFAZATROM

This drug, which is primarily used to prevent the clotting of blood, was used in a clinical trial on patients with advanced cancer and proved to be a powerful **inhibitor of tumor metastasis** (J.F. O'Donnell, American Journal of Clinical Oncology, 1986).

Nafazatrom does not affect the primary tumor. It does not inhibit tumor growth, nor cause a remission. The drug is well tolerated and several trials have confirmed its limited use (R.J. Warrell, et al., Cancer, 1986 and G.N. Hortobagyi, et al., Investigational New Drugs, 1986).

The method by which metastases are inhibited is apparently due to the anti-thrombotic effect (C.A. Maniglia, Journal of the National Cancer Institute, 1986).

****

ASPIRIN

Although aspirin is a synthetic drug, the substance on which it is based is derived from the white willow bark and its use dates back to the time of Hippocrates. In recent years, aspirin has received considerable notoriety in that it has been recommended for the prevention of heart attacks in small doses.

A. I. Popov, in 1987, reported in Medical Radiology (Moscow) that **aspirin** in combination with the B vitamin, **Niacin,** improved the five year survival time and reduced the recurrences of **bladder cancer** patients.

L. Rosenberg in the Journal of the National Cancer Institute in 1991, and G. Kune in Cancer, 1988, conducted large studies which indicated aspirin reduced the incidence of **colon cancer** and possibly **rectal cancer.**

A. Paganini-Hill, in a study of the elderly in California, indicated a slight increase in colon cancer. Howerver, The American Cancer Society conducted a study on over six hundred and sixty thousand people which indicated that there was more than a 40% reduction in the incidence of **colon and rectal cancer.**

Although aspirin is widely used, it is responsible for thousands of deaths each year, primarily through bleeding. In the discussion of Laetrile (Amygdalin) in this book, an interesting parallel between aspirin and laetrile is shown. Although the establishment may be correct in the anticoagulant effect being responsible for its anticancer action, the partial "laetrile" effect may be even more important. **I'll take laetrile, however, it's safer!**

****

FLUTAMIDE

National Cancer Institute studies indicate that flutamide is useful in the treatment of **prostate cancer.** Although it is used in combination with castration, it would certainly be preferable to take it on its own for individuals who wish to maintain a sexual life. It works by blocking the body's absorption of male hormones, some of which stimulate the growth of prostate cancer cells (R. N. Brogden, 1991). In **advanced cancers,** I do believe, flutamide has its place. However, local heat applied to the prostate and other therapies (see specific cancer therapy section) would be my choice.

****
MEGACE

Originally used as an oral contraceptive since 1959, and then as a treatment for **metastatic breast cancer,** megace is currently being used to **prevent weight loss** in cancer patients (R. Gorter, Oncology, 1991).

Tchekmedyian has done several studies on the use of megace in preventing cachexia or wasting (JAMA, 1987).

Patients experienced an increased sense of well-being, improved appetite and weight gain without significant toxicity (C.L. Loprinzi, Journal of the National Cancer Institute, 1990).

A notable study by S. A. Beck and M. J. Tisdale published in the British Journal of Cancer, showed that the use of megace in tumorous rats, resulted in increased appetite and prevention of weight loss. However, the major part of the weight loss consisted of water and there was a significant increase in the weight of the tumor. Their opinion was: increasing appetite and a gain in weight, were **not** sufficient reasons for using megace. I agree!

TAMOXIFEN

Since 1977, tamoxifen, a synthetic hormone, has been used as a treatment for **breast cancer.** It is currently being used for women whose breast cancers are **"estrogen receptor positive".**

S.S. Acktar, in 1991, reported in the European Journal of Surgical Oncology, that the use of tamoxifen negates the need for surgery in a large number of cases of breast cancer.

R. Wittes indicated in the Manual of Oncologic Therapeutics, 1992, that tamoxifen improved the effectiveness of L-PAM and 5-FU (chemotherapeutic agents).

M. Andersson, in the Journal of the National Cancer Institute, 1991, reported on a huge study showing that tamoxifen lessened the cancer incidence when used in conjunction with radiotherapy, but did not protect against the occurrence of cancer in the opposite breast. **However, concern was raised because of an**

elevated risk of endometrial cancer.

Other studies have indicated that tamoxifen can act as a **tumor promoter of liver cancer** in rats. This was confirmed by J.D. Yager and Y.E. Shi in Preventive Medicine, 1991. It should be noted that the risks and side effects of tamoxifen are being noted in more and more articles, appearing in Journals. The risks include eye damage, vasomotor (flushing) symptoms, cardiovascular damage and other major side effects. I would consider tamoxifen in the **"last resort"** category or **not at all.**

****

THIOPROLINE

Thioproline was discovered in 1937, but only in the last ten to twelve years has it been used as a treatment for cancer. The various reports which have appeared in journals are somewhat conflicting. It does not appear to be a truly effective drug and it has to be used for long periods of time. Its major use appears to be most successful in the treatment of skin cancers, especially those that metastasize and its major role seems to be in the prevention of reoccurrence of tumors. This information was provided by studies done by R.L. Grier, and reported in the Journal of Veterinary Research in 1984.

In 1989, J.F. Xie, of China, did a study which indicated a reversal of tumor tissue to normal after treatment with Thioproline. Although promising studies appeared in Spain, they could not be reproduced by other investigators (M. Gosalves, Bio. Med. Pharmacotherapy, 1982).

****

Chapter 16

Therapeutic Programs For Specific Cancers-

You Might Consider First.

IMPORTANT GENERAL ADVICE THAT APPLIES TO ALL CANCER THERAPY

The cornerstone for achieving optimal health or for reversing the cancer process is DIET. For this reason I have chosen the BUDWIG DIET as the goal to be achieved. The closer you follow it, the better the chances are for success.

Many of the recommendations for cancer prevention and therapy are simply foods. If the particular protocol you seek has a large number of items, do not let the years of establishment brainwashing confuse you. for most of them are natural foods, herbs and spices. Rather than thinking or using them like medicines, remember that they are really a part of your daily menu and their cost becomes part of your food budget ...

For example: Spices and herbs can be used for seasoning. The important mushrooms such as kombucha, maitake, shiitake and reishi are vegetables that go well with turkey, fish and with other vegetables. The beverage can be the Essaic formula, green tea, Chapparal, Pau D'Arco etc.

Note: DMSO is used in intravenous infusions of Amygdalin (Laetrile) and therefore is not listed separately.

BLADDER CANCER

- BUDWIG DIET (LINSEED OIL)
- CHELATION THERAPY
- AMYGDALIN (LAETRILE)
- OZONE THERAPY
- CRYOGENIC CELL INJECTIONS
- 714-X
- GLYOXIDE
- PROTEOLYTIC ENZYMES
- RECTAL COFFEE INSTILLATION
- COLONIC CLEANSING
- POSITIVE MIND-SPIRITUAL SUPPORT

THERAPEUTIC VITAMIN-MINERALS
(PLUS ADDITIONAL MEGADOSES AS SPECIFIED)

ADDITIONAL THERAPIES

Aspirin	BCG	Beta-Carotene
Vitamins	Vitamin K	Selenium
Evening-	Methylene-	MTH-68
Primrose	Blue	Kampo

SEE DOUBLE (**) AND SINGLE (*) STARS IN TABLE OF CONTENTS.

****

BRAIN CANCER

- **BUDWIG DIET (LINSEED OIL)**
- **CHELATION THERAPY**
- **AMYGDALIN (LAETRILE)**
- **OZONE THERAPY**
- **CRYOGENIC CELL INJECTIONS**
- **714-X**
- **GLYOXIDE**
- **PROTEOLYTIC ENZYMES**
- **RECTAL COFFEE INSTILLATION**
- **COLONIC CLEANSING**
- **POSITIVE MIND-SPIRITUAL SUPPORT**

THERAPEUTIC VITAMIN MINERAL
(PLUS ADDITIONAL MEGADOSES AS SPECIFIED)

ADDITIONAL THERAPIES

Antineoplastons	Arginine	Chaparral
Heat Therapy	Hydrazine	

SEE DOUBLE (**) AND SINGLE (*) STARS IN TABLE OF CONTENTS

****

BREAST CANCER

- ● BUDWIG DIET (LINSEED OIL)
- ● CHELATION THERAPY
- ● AMYGDALIN (LAETRILE)
- ● OZONE THERAPY
- ● CRYOGENIC CELL INJECTIONS
- ● 714-X
- ● GLYOXIDE
- ● PROTEOLYTIC ENZYMES
- ● RECTAL COFFEE INSTILLATION
- ● COLONIC CLEANSING
- ● POSITIVE MIND-SPIRITUAL SUPPORT

THERAPEUTIC VITAMIN-MINERALS
(PLUS ADDITIONAL MEGADOSES AS SPECIFIED)

ADDITIONAL THERAPIES

Algae	Ayur-Veda	Benzaldehyde
Beta-Carotene	Calcium	Canthaxanthin
Coley's Toxins	Electric Therapy	Fiber
Fish Oil	Garlic	Gossypol
Heat Therapy	Hydrazine	Indoles
Iscador	Lentinan	Magnesium
Megace	Molybdenum	MTH-68
Mushroom	Seaweed	Selenium
SOD	Staphage Lysate	Suramin
Tamoxifen	Thioproline	Vitamin C,
Cesium &		D, E and K
Rubidium		

SEE DOUBLE (**) AND SINGLE (*) STARS IN TABLE OF
CONTENTS

COLON\RECTAL CANCER

- BUDWIG DIET (LINSEED OIL)
- CHELATION THERAPY
- AMYGDALIN (LAETRILE)
- OZONE THERAPY
- CRYOGENIC CELL INJECTIONS
- 714-X
- GLYOXIDE
- PROTEOLYTIC ENZYMES
- RECTAL COFFEE INSTILLATION
- COLONIC CLEANSING
- POSITIVE MIND-SPIRITUAL SUPPORT

THERAPEUTIC VITAMIN MINERAL
(PLUS ADDITIONAL MEGADOSES AS SPECIFIED)

ADDITIONAL THERAPIES

Aspirin	Bestatin	Beta-Carotene
Calcium	Sulindac	Fiber
Fish Oil	Gerson	Phototherapy
Indoles	Krestin	Lactobacilli
Lentinan	Levamisole	Linseed Oil
Macrobiotic	MTH-68	Selenium
Vitamin A	Vitamin C	Vitamin D
Vitamin K	Cesium &	Calorie
	Rubidium	Balance

SEE DOUBLE (**) AND SINGLE (*) STARS IN TABLE OF CONTENTS

****

ESOPHAGEAL CANCER

- BUDWIG DIET (LINSEED OIL)
- CHELATION THERAPY
- AMYGDALIN (LAETRILE)
- OZONE THERAPY
- CRYOGENIC CELL INJECTIONS
- 714-X
- GLYOXIDE
- PROTEOLYTIC ENZYMES
- RECTAL COFFEE INSTILLATION
- COLONIC CLEANSING
- POSITIVE MIND-SPIRITUAL SUPPORT

THERAPEUTIC VITAMIN MINERAL
(PLUS ADDITIONAL MEGADOSES AS SPECIFIED)

ADDITIONAL THERAPIES

B Vitamins   Chinese Herbs   Molybdenum
Vitamin C

SEE DOUBLE (**) AND SINGLE (*) STARS IN TABLE OF
CONTENTS

****

HEAD & NECK CANCER

- BUDWIG DIET (LINSEED OIL)
- CHELATION THERAPY
- AMYGDALIN (LAETRILE)
- OZONE THERAPY
- CRYOGENIC CELL INJECTIONS
- 714-X
- GLYOXIDE
- PROTEOLYTIC ENZYMES
- RECTAL COFFEE INSTILLATION
- COLONIC CLEANSING
- POSITIVE MIND-SPIRITUAL SUPPORT

THERAPEUTIC VITAMIN MINERAL
(PLUS ADDITIONAL MEGADOSES AS SPECIFIED)

ADDITIONAL THERAPIES

Beta-Carotene	Heat Therapy	Phototherapy
Urea	Vitamin A	

SEE DOUBLE (**) AND SINGLE (*) STARS IN TABLE OF CONTENTS

****

THE CANCER SOLUTION

HUMAN IMMUNE DEFICIENCY RELATED
CANCERS (Related to the type of drugs being used)

- ● BUDWIG DIET (LINSEED OIL)
- ● CHELATION THERAPY
- ● AMYGDALIN (LAETRILE)
- ● OZONE THERAPY
- ● CRYOGENIC CELL INJECTIONS
- ● 714-X
- ● GLYOXIDE
- ● PROTEOLYTIC ENZYMES
- ● RECTAL COFFEE INSTILLATION
- ● COLONIC CLEANSING
- ● POSITIVE MIND-SPIRITUAL SUPPORT

THERAPEUTIC VITAMIN-MINERALS
(PLUS ADDITIONAL MEGADOSES AS SPECIFIED)

ADDITIONAL THERAPIES

Antineoplastons	Bestatin	Garlic
Germanium	Inosine	Megace
Monoclonals	Mushroom	Pau D'arco
Phototherapy	Seaweed	Shark
Cartilage	Tagamet	Vitamin C
Coley's Toxins	Thymic Factors	

SEE DOUBLE (**) AND SINGLE (*) STARS IN TABLE OF
CONTENTS

****

KIDNEY CANCER

- **BUDWIG DIET (LINSEED OIL)**
- **CHELATION THERAPY**
- **AMYGDALIN (LAETRILE)**
- **OZONE THERAPY**
- **CRYOGENIC CELL INJECTIONS**
- **714-X**
- **GLYOXIDE**
- **PROTEOLYTIC ENZYMES**
- **RECTAL COFFEE INSTILLATION**
- **COLONIC CLEANSING**
- **POSITIVE MIND-SPIRITUAL SUPPORT**

THERAPEUTIC VITAMIN MINERAL
(PLUS ADDITIONAL MEGADOSES AS SPECIFIED)

ADDITIONAL THERAPIES

Arginine	Bryostatins	Onconase
Suramin	Tamoxifen	Vitamin C
Vitamin K		

SEE DOUBLE (**) AND SINGLE (*) STARS IN TABLE OF
CONTENTS

****

LEUKEMIA

- BUDWIG DIET (LINSEED OIL)
- CHELATION THERAPY
- AMYGDALIN (LAETRILE)
- OZONE THERAPY
- CRYOGENIC CELL INJECTIONS
- 714-X
- GLYOXIDE
- PROTEOLYTIC ENZYMES
- RECTAL COFFEE INSTILLATION
- COLONIC CLEANSING
- POSITIVE MIND-SPIRITUAL SUPPORT

THERAPEUTIC VITAMIN MINERAL
(PLUS ADDITIONAL MEGADOSES AS SPECIFIED)

ADDITIONAL THERAPIES

Algae	Bestatin	Bryostatins
Butyric Acid	Chaparral	CSF
DMSO	Enzymes	Gossypol
Evening Primrose	Hydrazine	Krestin
Lactobacilli	Methylene Blue	Monoclonals
Phototherapy	Seaweed	Selenium
Vitamin C	Vitamin D	Vitamin K

SEE DOUBLE (**) AND SINGLE (*) STARS IN TABLE OF CONTENTS

****

LIVER CANCER

- **BUDWIG DIET (LINSEED OIL)**
- **CHELATION THERAPY**
- **AMYGDALIN (LAETRILE)**
- **OZONE THERAPY**
- **CRYOGENIC CELL INJECTIONS**
- **714-X**
- **GLYOXIDE**
- **PROTEOLYTIC ENZYMES**
- **RECTAL COFFEE INSTILLATION**
- **COLONIC CLEANSING**
- **POSITIVE MIND-SPIRITUAL SUPPORT**

THERAPEUTIC VITAMIN-MINERALS
(PLUS ADDITIONAL MEGADOSES AS SPECIFIED)

ADDITIONAL THERAPIES

Arginine	Green Tea	Lentinan
Selenium	Tagamet	Urea
Vitamin K	Cesium &	Coley's
Evening Primrose	Rubidium	Toxins

SEE DOUBLE (**) AND SINGLE (*) STARS IN TABLE OF CONTENTS

****

LUNG CANCER

- **BUDWIG DIET (LINSEED OIL)**
- **CHELATION THERAPY**
- **AMYGDALIN (LAETRILE)**
- **OZONE THERAPY**
- **CRYOGENIC CELL INJECTIONS**
- **714-X**
- **GLYOXIDE**
- **PROTEOLYTIC ENZYMES**
- **RECTAL COFFEE INSTILLATION**
- **COLONIC CLEANSING**
- **POSITIVE MIND-SPIRITUAL SUPPORT**

THERAPEUTIC VITAMIN MINERAL
(PLUS ADDITIONAL MEGADOSES AS SPECIFIED)

ADDITIONAL THERAPIES

Ayur-Veda	BCG	Bestatin
Beta-Carotene	B Vitamins	Urea
Chinese Herbs	Ellagic Acid	Green Tea
Gerson Therapy	Hydrazine	Iscador
Muroctasin Mushroom	Phototherapy	Seaweed
Thymic Factors	SOD	Vitamin A
Vitamin C	Vitamin E	Vitamin K
Cesium & Rubidium		

SEE DOUBLE (**) AND SINGLE (*) STARS IN TABLE OF
CONTENTS

****

LYMPHOMA

- ● BUDWIG DIET (LINSEED OIL)
- ● CHELATION THERAPY
- ● AMYGDALIN (LAETRILE)
- ● OZONE THERAPY
- ● CRYOGENIC CELL INJECTIONS
- ● 714-X
- ● GLYOXIDE
- ● PROTEOLYTIC ENZYMES
- ● RECTAL COFFEE INSTILLATION
- ● COLONIC CLEANSING
- ● POSITIVE MIND-SPIRITUAL SUPPORT

THERAPEUTIC VITAMIN MINERAL
(PLUS ADDITIONAL MEGADOSES AS SPECIFIED)

ADDITIONAL THERAPIES

Bestatin	Coley's Toxins	Hydrazine
Monoclonals	Phototherapy	Splenopentin
Tagamet	Vitamin A	Cesium & Rubidium

SEE DOUBLE (**) AND SINGLE (*) STARS IN TABLE OF CONTENTS

****

MELANOMA (see SKIN)

****

ORAL CANCER

- **BUDWIG DIET (LINSEED OIL)**
- **CHELATION THERAPY**
- **AMYGDALIN (LAETRILE)**
- **OZONE THERAPY**
- **CRYOGENIC CELL INJECTIONS**
- **714-X**
- **GLYOXIDE**
- **PROTEOLYTIC ENZYMES**
- **RECTAL COFFEE INSTILLATION**
- **COLONIC CLEANSING**
- **POSITIVE MIND-SPIRITUAL SUPPORT**

THERAPEUTIC VITAMIN MINERAL
(PLUS ADDITIONAL MEGADOSES AS SPECIFIED)

ADDITIONAL THERAPIES

Beta-Carotene	Selenium	Thioproline
Vitamin A	Vitamin C	

SEE DOUBLE (**) AND SINGLE (*) STARS IN TABLE OF CONTENTS

****

PANCREATIC CANCER

- **BUDWIG DIET (LINSEED OIL)**
- **CHELATION THERAPY**
- **AMYGDALIN (LAETRILE)**
- **OZONE THERAPY**
- **CRYOGENIC CELL INJECTIONS**
- **714-X**
- **GLYOXIDE**
- **PROTEOLYTIC ENZYMES**
- **RECTAL COFFEE INSTILLATION**
- **COLONIC CLEANSING**
- **POSITIVE MIND-SPIRITUAL SUPPORT**

THERAPEUTIC VITAMIN-MINERALS
(PLUS ADDITIONAL MEGADOSES AS SPECIFIED)

ADDITIONAL THERAPIES

Cesium & Rubidium	Fish Oil Onconase	Gossypol Vitamin C

SEE DOUBLE (**) AND SINGLE (*) STARS IN TABLE OF CONTENTS

****

PROSTATE CANCER

- BUDWIG DIET (LINSEED OIL)
- CHELATION THERAPY
- AMYGDALIN (LAETRILE)
- OZONE THERAPY
- CRYOGENIC CELL INJECTIONS
- 714-X
- GLYOXIDE
- PROTEOLYTIC ENZYMES
- RECTAL COFFEE INSTILLATION
- COLONIC CLEANSING
- POSITIVE MIND-SPIRITUAL SUPPORT

THERAPEUTIC VITAMIN-MINERALS
(PLUS ADDITIONAL MEGADOSES AS SPECIFIED)

ADDITIONAL THERAPIES

Heat Therapy	Indoles	Kampo
MTH-68	Selenium	Suramin
Vitamin A	Zinc	Cesium & Rubidium

SEE DOUBLE (**) AND SINGLE (*) STARS IN TABLE OF CONTENTS

****

RECTAL CANCER
(see COLON)

****

SKIN CANCER
(MELANOMA INCLUDED)

- **BUDWIG DIET (LINSEED OIL)**
- **CHELATION THERAPY**
- **AMYGDALIN (LAETRILE)**
- **OZONE THERAPY**
- **CRYOGENIC CELL INJECTIONS**
- **714-X**
- **GLYOXIDE**
- **PROTEOLYTIC ENZYMES**
- **RECTAL COFFEE INSTILLATION**
- **COLONIC CLEANSING**
- **POSITIVE MIND-SPIRITUAL SUPPORT**

THERAPEUTIC VITAMIN-MINERALS
(PLUS ADDITIONAL MEGADOSES AS SPECIFIED)

ADDITIONAL THERAPIES

Astragalus	Azelaic Acid	B Vitamins
Chaparral	Garlic	Green Tea
Hydrazine	Inosine	Kampo
Monoclonals	MTH-68	Selenium
Spices	Thymic Factors	Vitamin A
BCG Bestatin	Vitamin C	Vitamin D
Coley's Toxins	Heat Therapy	Tagamet

Hoxsey (or Mohs) Salve (Zinc Chloride, Antimony Tri-sulfide and Bloodroot)

SEE DOUBLE (**) AND SINGLE (*) STARS IN TABLE OF CONTENTS

****

STOMACH CANCER

- **BUDWIG DIET (LINSEED OIL)**
- **CHELATION THERAPY**
- **AMYGDALIN (LAETRILE)**
- **OZONE THERAPY**
- **CRYOGENIC CELL INJECTIONS**
- **714-X**
- **GLYOXIDE**
- **PROTEOLYTIC ENZYMES**
- **RECTAL COFFEE INSTILLATION**
- **COLONIC CLEANSING**
- **POSITIVE MIND-SPIRITUAL SUPPORT**

THERAPEUTIC VITAMIN-MINERALS
(PLUS ADDITIONAL MEGADOSES AS SPECIFIED)

ADDITIONAL THERAPIES

Benzaldehyde	Bioflavonoids	Green Tea
Hydrazine	Indoles	Krestin
Lentinan	Molybdenum	MTH-68
Selenium	SOD	Spices
Vitamin A	Vitamin C	Vitamin E

SEE DOUBLE (**) AND SINGLE (*) STARS IN TABLE OF CONTENTS

****

TESTICULAR CANCER

- **BUDWIG DIET (LINSEED OIL)**
- **CHELATION THERAPY**
- **AMYGDALIN (LAETRILE)**
- **OZONE THERAPY**
- **CRYOGENIC CELL INJECTIONS**
- **714-X**
- **GLYOXIDE**
- **PROTEOLYTIC ENZYMES**
- **RECTAL COFFEE INSTILLATION**
- **COLONIC CLEANSING**
- **POSITIVE MIND-SPIRITUAL SUPPORT**

THERAPEUTIC VITAMIN-MINERALS
(PLUS ADDITIONAL MEGADOSES AS SPECIFIED)

ADDITIONAL THERAPIES

Maruyama Vaccine   Gossypol   Megace

SEE DOUBLE (**) AND SINGLE (*) STARS IN TABLE OF CONTENTS

****

Chapter 17

Very Interesting!
What's Going On?

Jon Rappoprt, the author of "The AIDS Myth" sent me a letter reference to my book on AIDS, *"The Ultimate Deception"*. In it he included two cards with health information distributed free by a group called In Your Face, a division of People for a Free America - "We are not right wing or left wing or moderate. We're real. Make copies and pass it on." So ... I thought it would be the right thing for me to pass it on ...

WHAT IS HEALTH?

1. Every year in the U.S. 60,000 people die as a result of unnecessary surgery.
2. 15 million unneeded surgeries are performed annually.
3. Of these operations, 350,000 are unnecessary Caesareans.
4. 1 million citizens are suffering from brain damage as a result of the administration of one class of psychiatric drugs - the neuroleptics.
5. 800,000 American school children are prescribed a cheap form of speed called Ritalin. This drug is given for a bogus condition called ADD (Attention Deficit Disorder). Ritalin eventually causes hyperactivity and depression. It can cause acute withdrawal symptoms, and an amphetamine-like psychosis. **Ritalin makes drug addicts.**
6. There is now compelling evidence that, for 70-80% of the

214

cancers that kill people, **chemotherapy is completely ineffective and does not improve the quality of life. Chemotherapy is cancer-causing** and kills human cells indiscriminately.

7. AZT, the central drug prescribed for AIDS, terminates DNA synthesis in the body. It also attacks the bone marrow, where immune-system cells are manufactured, and so creates the symptoms of AIDS.

8. In order for all of the above to be ushered in, literally thousands of drug-studies had to be approved by the FDA, the agency which licenses all medical drugs. We are talking about major felonies, at least on the order of negligent homicide.

*** Authors comment: AZT causes AIDS! - See
"The Ultimate Deception" - can be ordered from
Peltec Publishing Co., Inc.
4400 N. Federal Hwy., Suite 210
Boca Raton, FL 33431
Tel. 1 800 214-3645**

SEE:

1. Chemotherapy of Advanced Epithelial Cancer, Ulrich Abel, Hippokrates Verlag Stuttgart, 1990. An English translation is available from People Against Cancer, P.O. Box 10, Otho, Iowa, 50569.

2. Poison by Prescription: The AZT Story, John Lauritsen, Asklepios, 1990.

3. The Profits of Misery: How Inpatient Psychiatric Treatment Bilks the System and Betrays Our Trust. Hearing before Select Committee on Children, Youth and Families, House of Representatives, April 28, 1992. U.S. Government Printing Office.

4. Mass Murderers in White Coats: Psychiatric Genocide in Nazi Germany and the United States, Lenny Lapon 1986, Psychiatric Genocide Research Institute, 55 Bryant Street, Springfield, MA 01108.

5. Toxic Psychiatry, Peter Breggins, St. Martin's Press 1991.

INFORMATION FOR SURVIVAL
- IT'S PERSONAL

For your health and your children's health:

1. Demand and buy organically grown fruits, vegetables and grains. Don't eat food sauced with pesticides.
2. Don't take pharmaceutical drugs. Exception: You really have an acute crisis and feel you must. Then do so only long enough to bring yourself back to square one. From that point, rebuild your health naturally.
3. Don't eat meat. Don't eat beef, chicken fish, pork, lamb, cheese, eggs, milk products. *
4. Realize that a diet of whole grains, fruits and vegetables is even recommended by a number of orthodox researchers as the healthiest.
5. Doing all of the above is more than personal. It's political. If you're interested, turn this card over and read the fine print.

* I make exceptions as indicated elsewhere - small portions (3 oz.) 3 - 4 times a week.

IT'S POLITICAL

1. The 8 biggest pesticide companies in the world are also drug companies. Among them, they own a very large share of North American seed companies.
2. The Big 8 are: Bayer, Dupont, Dow/Elanco, Monsanto, Ciba-Geigy, Rhone-Poulenc, ICI, and Hoechst.
3. They are currently inserting special genes in their seeds. Purpose? To allow these seeds to grow into food crops which will absorb more pesticides than ever without curling up and dying.
4. This means that you will be eating more poison. The soil will be drenched with more poison. The Big 8 will be making more money selling pesticides to farmers.
5. The Big 8 and other huge companies, like them also make highly toxic drugs (and hormones and antibiotics for farm

animals). For instance, Rhone-Poulenc and Dupont make Thorazine and Moban, two psychiatric compounds called neuroleptics. All neuroleptics can and do cause brain damage. It is estimated that in the U.S., one million people have suffered brain damage from the 20 or so neuroleptic drugs on the market. This is the biggest medically induced plague in history.

6. Ciba-Geigy makes Ritalin, a form of speed given to upwards of 800,000 school children in America diagnosed with a bogus syndrome called Attention Deficit Disorder. This drug is addicting and can cause hyperactivity and even an amphetamine-like psychosis. This is called Manufacturing Addicts in School.

7. ICI makes Elavil, an antidepressant. Typical antidepressants sedate the user, cause withdrawal symptoms, blur the vision, and repress the working of the gut, bladder, and sexual organs.

8. Dow makes Prozac, a hot-selling antidepressant that has been linked to suicidal and murderous behaviors.

9. IF YOU FOLLOW THE IDEAS ON SIDE ONE OF THIS CARD, YOU NOT ONLY IMPROVE YOUR OWN HEALTH, YOU STOP BUYING WHAT THESE CORPORATE GIANTS ARE SELLING. IF ENOUGH PEOPLE DO THIS, THESE COMPANIES GO BROKE, STRANGER THINGS HAVE HAPPENED. THIS IS NOT A BOYCOTT DONE TO GET PRESS COVERAGE. THIS IS FOREVER.

****

DEADLY DIETS - WHAT THE HELL HAVE WE BEEN EATING?

When prescribing a diet for my patients, lecturing to professionals and the public, or even in a casual discussion at a gathering, I have frequently heard the comment; "With everything that you say is bad for us, it doesn't seem as if there's anything left for us to eat!" To a degree that is true. However, if we remember that the effect of a poison is dose related, then the objective is to minimize the danger as much as possible. It is virtually impossible to eliminate all the factors that pose a hazard to our health. It is rather easy however, to reduce the threat to a level that can be dispensed with readily by our natural defenses. It is important to become familiar with the most common and dangerous foods and additives, and the problems created in the preparation of food. There are not that many things to remember. Once you are familiar with the basic foods that protect you the most, a smattering of the undesirable are not likely to put your health at risk.

As I mentioned before, it has been estimated that we can consume harmful compounds when eating a charcoal broiled steak equal to smoking 600 cigarettes. Coal tars have long been known to be carcinogenic not only to the lungs but to the skin as well. This problem in broiling meat can be remedied if the flame or source of heat is above the meat thus allowing the fat to drip out of the meat and on to the pan. In this way the fat is not heated to excessive degrees and does not burn into the meat. I prefer gas or electric heat because using a microwave to avoid the formation of carcinogens results in the change of the molecular structure of the meat and alters its nutritional qualities. Additional protection is given if green vegetables are eaten in the same meal. The amount of mutagenic substances excreted in the urine are significantly decreased. This is further evidence that green vegetables provide protection against cancer. The chapter dealing with linseed oil discusses at length how this remarkable oil provides additional protection against many of the foods which are processed and refined thus contributing to the development of cancer. Therefore, supplementing a meal that has steak as the main item with a vegetable salad and a linseed oil dressing would give you maximum protection from the harmful affects.

It is not surprising, however, that when obvious and serious dangers to the public are exposed in which profits are involved, very little is done. As you will read elsewhere in this book, one of the greatest dangers to the public health and welfare is the food industry. **When the World Health Organization, in 1977, issued a notice to the nations of the world that processed oils used in the cooking and preparation of foods were a great danger to the health of all peoples, and even advocated legal action against the production of such oils, not even one nation took steps to outlaw their use.**

I abhor Government control. However, regulating and

controlling the production of deadly substances is not the same as telling us what we can or cannot eat. The same FDA which **restricts** information about the therapeutic powers of various herbs, vitamins and minerals, **allows** carcinogenic poisons, such as processed oils to remain on the shelves. Although it is important to stress those foods we should include in our diet, it is equally important to point out those foods and eating habits which should be avoided. They play a direct role in the causation of all diseases, including cancer. The following are substances which must be eliminated from the diet if you wish to achieve maximum health and prevent most diseases including cancer. Some are discussed at greater length in other chapters of this book.

Processed Fats and Oils

Avoid completely all fats and oils that have been processed. The only safe products are those which are **cold-pressed, unprocessed and fresh.** If you see the words hydrogenated or partially hydrogenated, avoid these foods at all costs.

Excessive Dietary Fat

A diet rich in vegetables and low in fat, i.e. as eaten by Seventh Day Adventists and Mormons, decreases the risk of colon, breast and prostate cancers. If, in addition, tobacco, alcohol and caffienated beverages are eliminated, the risk of breast, ovarian, urinary, or blood cancers are also diminished. The type of fat (saturated or unsaturated) consumed in the diet does not appear to be that important. It is the total amount of fat. This is because all fats eaten in the diet are converted to carcinogens by cooking or processing. The demand on digestive processes may damage the intestinal wall thus increasing susceptibility to carcinogens. I strongly suggest that the intake of natural fats in our diet, should be limited to approximately fifteen to twenty percent of our total caloric intake. It is recommended by the establishment, that the total intake of fat be held down to less than 30% of the day's calories. Do you need more incentive to change? Well consider this:

When the Japanese, who eat a low fat diet, move to the

U.S. and change their eating habits, colon and breast cancer increases markedly. The American cancer death rate is 5 to 10 times higher than in Japan.

Total Caloric Intake

The incidence of almost every disease is increased in individuals who are overweight. **For example, the excess weight** stimulates an increase in estrogen which increases certain tumor growth. You now know it is possible to eat and be fully satisfied and never go hungry with a healthy diet and yet, maintain your weight at a healthy level.

Protein Intake from all types of Fish and Meat

Unfortunately deadly metals like mercury and other industrial poisons are contaminating the waters of the planet. Our cattle are laced with hormones, antibiotics, pesticides etc. Free range are the safest, but not entirely. Keep it to a minimum - small portions (3-4 oz., three to four times a week)

Chemicals and Preservatives in Food

Avoid anything that you cannot pronounce. Beware of all preservatives, colorings and substances that were not created by "God".

Foods that are overheated, gassed or irradiated

Especially avoid processed foods containing nitrates and nitrites. Foods that have been smoked. Foods that have been sprayed with pesticides and herbicides. Coffee, tea and tobacco.

Fats would not normally be such a problem in our diet if we did not have so many foods which are processed and foods to which fats are added. The natural fats found in foods are extremely healthy for us and necessary. Cholesterol has been singled out frequently because of its association with coronary artery disease, usually generalized as atherosclerosis. However, it is not the total intake of cholesterol which poses the real danger, it is the fact that we are eating processed oils which causes the cholesterol to precipitate out and become "gummy". It then adheres to the walls of arteries and, along with calcium and other minerals, form plaque. Contrary to what you have read, eating eggs, natural cheese, butter and milk in moderate amounts, actually provide protection rather than harm.

Our bodies naturally produce cholesterol. Without cholesterol, we would not have any hormones. You have probably read about the high density lipo-proteins as being protective. It is this type of fatty acid substance that helps keep cholesterol in solution in the blood. Because of the processing of oils and the creation of artificial fatty substances, such as margarine, our diets are almost devoid of these natural fatty acids. When fats are processed, poisonous solvents, such as carbon tetrachloride are used to extract oil. The oil is heated and mixed with lye, formaldehyde and other chemicals. Important ingredients are filtered out. These foods are then altered by hydrogenation and then chemicals are added to extend the shelf life. What we are left with are foods which, as a species, we have not adapted to over the millions of years of our existence. These are no longer foods, they are partially usable poisons!

Foods that are "smoked"

Gastric cancer has been directly linked with the eating of smoked foods. Except for vegetables and fruits, almost every other food is now smoked and has become a part of the cuisine of the world. Hydrocarbons are absorbed during this process and have been long known to be carcinogenic. In addition, **many smoked foods are preserved with salt or nitrates which are also carcinogenic** and, therefore, become foods of double jeopardy. Occasional ingestion of these foods does not create a real problem, but when they become a frequent part of the diet, they are unquestionably of great danger. The popularity of barbecueing, with or without the barbecue sauce, is now world-wide. Unsuspecting families who frequently prepare meals out in the back yard, over a charcoal grill, are exposing their members to dangerous compounds. It warrants repeating and I know it sounds incredible, but eating one charcoaled broiled steak is equivalent to smoking thirty packs of cigarettes (600 cigarettes). The dangerous effects of hydrocarbons has been known for centuries. When you broil food over charcoal, the fat from that food drips onto the charcoal and produces smoke that contains carcinogens so at least stand upwind.

Processing of Foods

Recently, radiation of foods has become increasingly popular with manufacturers and food processors. It can now be added to the long list of processes which change the actual cellular structure of foods, robbing them of their natural nutrition and converting them into compounds which are actually carcinogenic. Foods that have been roasted, browned, cooked, gassed, irradiated, chemically treated and hydrogenated are all substantially changed from their normal state. In hospitals, where milk from the mother's breast is stored in the refrigerators for the new born infant to have while the mother is resting, is then re-heated by microwave. It has been proven that microwaving of the mother's milk, robs it of all the protective nutrients that are necessary for a baby's survival. In all of these forms of processing, substances called mutagens are formed and they have the ability to cause mutations in genetic structure.

Foods prepared in fast-food restaurants, particularly hamburgers, roasted coffee, and most commercially processed foods were shown by Barry Commoner, at the Centre for Biology of Natural Substances, Washington University, to cause the development of these mutagens. He showed that foods cooked at high temperatures (300 degrees Fahrenheit) develop carcinogenic substances.

When broiling meat, the best way to do this is with a flame above the meat. That way the fat can drip into the pan, will not smoke and cause hydrocarbons to form. I do not advocate the use of a microwave for cooking any foods. It has been determined that eating green vegetables along with your meat, can reduce the sum of mutagenic substances formed. Particularly useful in this way are wheat sprouts, Brussels sprouts, cabbage, broccoli, spinach and lettuce, preferably not Iceberg lettuce.

Meat Protein

A conclusive study over a ten year period, involving hundreds of millions of Chinese, was performed by a Dr. Gun-Shuy Chen of Beijing and Dr. T. Colin Campbell of Cornell University, revealed powerful nutritional evidence that when a diet contained considerable meat protein, there was an increased incidence of colon/rectal cancer, of leukemia, cancer of the lungs, esophagus and stomach. Elevated serum cholesterol levels were correlated with positive tests for stomach, rectal, lung cancers and leukemia. The study also revealed that high intake of Vitamin A protected against cancer of the stomach and the esophagus. High Vitamin C intake also protected against stomach and esophageal cancers. High Beta-Carotene levels protected against stomach and esophageal cancers, as did elevated intake of selenium. High fiber intake resulted in a reduction in the occurrence of all cancer.

Tobacco and Alcohol

Tobacco and alcohol do not fall under the aegis of the food and drug administration in the United States. Although it is obvious that they are both drugs, they are protected from control by powerful economic interests. It is estimated that tobacco plays a role in thirty percent of all cancers. It is now generally accepted that it is the major contributing cause of lung cancer. Oral (mouth) and throat cancer are markedly increased (twice as much) in individuals who chew tobacco rather than smoking it, and the public is being made increasingly aware of the dangers of secondary smoke, is those who are breathing the air in close proximity to smokers.

Although it has generally been accepted for a long period of time that two drinks a day should be your limit in order to avoid damage to the liver and to other tissues of the body, recent information indicates that two drinks a week can do substantial damage to brain cells and to the liver. In addition, alcohol acts as a transport for substances that are carcinogenic and therefore promotes mutagens.

Cooking with aluminium ware, in recent year, has become suspect as a cause of Alzheimer's Disease. However, Dr. Barry Commoner also demonstrated that mutagens were formed when meat was prepared in metalware for long periods of time. Butter and cooking oils that are overheated, begin to smoke and they, too, cause carcinogens. What we consider normal cooking can actually produce mutagens in meat, fish, baked goods, cereals, toasted bread, French fried potatoes and caramel.

Cooking with a Chinese Wok or the Nouveau Cuisine of the French, reduce the overcooking of food and is far more healthy and a palatable way of preparing crisp vegetables and other foods.

Remember: Reducing or eliminating nitrite-cured, salt cured or smoked meats from the diet, reduces the risk of stomach and esophageal cancers. The addition of Vitamin C to the diet will reduce the amount of the nitrosamines manufactured by the body from nitrites. All beers and many whiskeys contain nitrosamines. Pickled foods are also high in nitrosamines.

****

COOKING METHODS

Avoid eating meats cooked at temperatures above 300 degrees F. Lightly steamed vegetables are preferred. Raw vegetables are even better. Avoid foods that are "blackened" by cooking (this includes bread that is toasted and butter that is blackened). Avoid processed oils. Use only cold pressed, raw oils if possible. Avoid fried foods completely. Addition of Vitamin C, Selenium and Vitamin E in the diet can aid in preventing carcinogenic changes. Eating green vegetables, such as spinach, cabbage, broccoli, mustard greens, brussel sprouts, lettuce and wheat sprouts, at the same time as other foods, also prevent carcinogenic changes. Alcohol increases the risk of liver cancer. Avoid over-ripe or mouldy foods. Avoid microwave cooking and irradiated foods. Avoid all food products that have been exposed to insecticides, hormones and antibiotics. Vitamin A reduces the risk of stomach and esophageal cancers. A protein-rich diet increases the risk of stomach and esophageal cancers. Selenium and Beta-carotene reduces the risk of esophageal and stomach cancer. A fiber-rich diet decreases the risk of all cancers. A low-fat, low-cholesterol diet is associated with a lower risk of stomach, colon, rectal and lung cancers, as well as leukemia.

****

GENERAL RULES TO FOLLOW

Increase the intake of fruits, vegetables, nuts and berries. Increase the intake of fiber-rich foods, such as vegetables and whole grains, as well as fruits. Eat raw foods whenever possible. Cooked foods are better if baked or steamed. Eat fish, preferably the cold water variety, several times a week. Eat poultry from free range farms and cook it well. Reduce meat intake; reduce salt intake; and substitute spices, herbs and lemon. Avoid all processed foods, especially foods containing processed oils. Avoid pickled, smoked or cured foods. Reduce or eliminate alcohol from your diet.

****

RISKY BUSINESS

There are many businesses which produce products and services that endanger the health and welfare of the public. Many of these are responsible for the development of many types of cancer, either directly or indirectly. Household insecticides and cleaners produce fumes which are highly toxic. Microwave cooking devices are now in millions of homes and alarms are present everywhere. University of Washington researchers in the Bio-electric research laboratory showed that cancers, particularly those of the endocrine system can be promoted by microwave and other forms of electro-magnetic radiation. **Tanning lamps produce ultra-violet A which ages skin (UV-A), and ultraviolet B (UV- B) which causes skin cancer.** The "innocent" computer monitor also poses a danger and I would strongly advise that anyone working in front of a computer for long periods of time, should use the new screens that eliminate even low levels of radiation.

****

DENTAL AMALGAM -
JUST A LITTLE BIT OF CANCER?

Last, but never to be omitted, are the teeth! On April 27, 1993, an article appeared in the New York Times in the Science Times section. It talked of a new suspect in the mystery of what causes resistance in microorganisms. The suspect is amalgam, the so-called "silver" fillings which are in reality 50% **mercury**, the most poisonous metal known to humans. It is reasoned by investigators that if mercury maintains a population of bacteria resistant to mercury, it might do the same with fostering their resistance to antibiotics. Dr. Anne O. Summers at the University of Georgia has demonstrated that this is what occurs in monkeys. The American Dental Association commented that animal studies "cannot be viewed as affecting humans"!!!! **I can't believe they said that!!!** Their use of the word "affecting", even if it's their mistake and not a typographical error, it is a good indication of their science. Let me tell you why I bring this up in a book on cancer:

BECAUSE MERCURY IS A *CARCINOGENIC* AS WELL AS A POISON!

In the article it is mentioned that studies have shown that the mercury slowly leaches out of the fillings. The ADA has staunchly defended the use of amalgam in spite of the fact that there is substantial evidence that patients with many serious illnesses, including psychotic episodes and deadly allergic responses, were cured by removing the amalgam. There are marvelous books and reams of articles dealing with amalgam's threat to health. It is my opinion that I would rather have a ceramic filling than being slowly poisoned by mercury. Not only that, if you have gold fillings in your mouth also, you effectively have a battery producing electrical current! Of course, the ADA says the evidence is not convincing and the amount is minute. My thoughts are that a little bit of poison and a little bit of cancer is like being a little bit pregnant! Besides doesn't the ADA know that the effect of drugs including poison is dose related and cumulative. The formula is: amount X no. of doses = toxicity!

Obviously, I believe in prevention, so I cannot leave you without a recommendation to help you avoid fillings in the first place. No microorganism can adapt to hydrogen peroxide (H2O2). Many dentists recommend 3% H2O2 as a gargle or rinse and making a paste along with baking soda (sodium bicarbonate). Three times a day is advised. It is great for dentures too!

Did I hear you ask, "What about the flouride?" My Opinion?

- AVOID FLUORIDE LIKE POISON! WHY? BECAUSE IT IS! NOT ONLY THAT, IT'S CARCINOGENIC!

FLOURIDE has never been proven to prevent tooth decay, it has been outlawed in many countries or sections of countries because the evidence is overwhelming that **FLOURIDE causes premature aging, slows DNA repair, irregular DNA synthesis and malignant transformation of cells (American Cancer Institute - 1963). DRINK BOTTLED WATER AND USE FLORIDE FREE TOOTHPASTE!**

****

Chapter 18

Parting Thoughts Of A Medical Heretic

The rights of the individual to exercise freedom of choice and to determine the care of their bodies and the course of their lives must be held inviolate. Medicine, above all, should always be mindful that in most diseases, especially chronic conditions, that the beneficial results of faith, the mind and healthy life practices, render insignificant any claims thus far made for drugs and other medical therapies. That, in truth, those positive results which the establishment condescendingly refers to as the "placebo effect", have a far better record of safety (obviously) and efficacy than we are willing to admit. The arrogance of the medical establishment and the hubris of many of physicians must give way to humility and open-mindedness. Serious consideration of all natural alternatives to our own, often destructive, drug culture, must be given top priority.

True science fosters all concepts to flourish in the marketplace of ideas and recognizes its own limitations. Claims, when possible, must be subject to scientific proof and be validated. The means to do this, has to be accomplished by private or government funds, carefully and scrupulously screening out any influence by the pharmaceutical industry political forces and the medical establishment. In areas where we have nothing better to offer, we should welcome any safe therapy that has produced positive results. We must put an end to the fantasies about questionable benefits which perpetuate the use of dangerous drugs and insane therapies of modern medicine. Benefits are often claimed that are grossly exaggerated or non-existent, many of which have already discredited the medical profession and the pharmaceutical industry.

How many more types of useless and hazardous drugs, surgeries and medical therapies will we have to abandon before we realize that we have become the victims of self-serving individuals and corporations.

Why are thousands of redundant journals paid for by the pharmaceutical industry? It is a simple case of brain-washing! Medicine's integrity, education and independence, as well as the welfare of the patients they claim to serve, would be better served by one-tenth that number of journals financed and scrutinized by truly independent physicians and scientists. The punishment for corruption and collusion on the part of anyone should be subjected to severe penalties and punishment. Most importantly, there must not be suppression of opposing views, monopoly of medical schools of thought or therapy by consensus.

The stories, many of them well-documented, of the often mysterious disappearance, confiscation and destruction of the scientific notes, clinical records, evidence and proof of the efficacy of medical scientific inventions and medical therapies, have been the subject of numerous books. Many have been recorded in the congressional record. The original work of Rife, Tessla, Cayce and many others have been have been partially or completely lost to us in these ways. Currently, the brilliant discoveries of some of our most honored and world-renowned scientists such as Linus Pauling and Peter Duesberg, have been subject to the worst kind of dishonest, corrupt, conniving, counterfeit and baseless personal and professional character assassination. To sue their attackers is often extremely difficult. Victims have often been rendered virtually penniless by the loss of position or grants. It is often impossible to find a competent attorney to take a solid case on contingency because the costs of preparation are so high.

Excellent and dedicated physicians, too many to mention, have lost their licences to practice or have been silenced by the pharmaceutical-medical-government complex. Most have been drained completely by the enormous expenses involved in legal defense, usually in administrative hearings and then have to fight again in a court of law. Corruption is rampant and practiced by administrative hearings. Doctrine is dictated by vested interests. The media, frequently owned by the very same corporations that stand to lose by the recognition of "alternative" and natural non-patentable remedies, present to the public an incredibly biased, distorted and incomplete point of few. Even advertisements for publications about alternative therapies are rejected. A barrier of silence exists, but worse, the press willingly prints any unfounded condemnation by the establishment of alternative therapies. Very rarely is any evidence provided, usually it is only the opinion of someone who has never used them. The press is eager to report some scientific discovery that is purported to someday lead to a cure for cancer or any one of a hundred chronic degenerative diseases. For cancer, that "someday" is already eighty years, and we're still waiting. Meanwhile, we are being duped into believing that the state of the art is to "cut, burn, or poison" with surgery, radiation and chemotherapy. There is substantial evidence that the patient would be better off doing nothing.

I am convinced from experience that many "alternative" therapies are effective and succeed where "orthodox" medicine fails. The difference in theory and philosophy is the major reason. It is often said that "the scientific method has been proven scientifically". The tragedies wrought by countless drugs, that were "proven effective" by the "scientifically established double-blind study", fill millions of graves. What is commonly referred to as "side-effects", are in truth, direct effects. Many "side-effects" are deadly. Doctors not only bury their mistakes, but also those of the drug industry.

Medicine operates under many theories that have never been proven. Raymond Peat, Ph.D., in his book, "Generative Energy: Protecting and Restoring The Wholeness of Life", comments; "The 'genetic defect' theory of disease holds the promise of a gene implant for every problem. Interestingly, the people who point out that 'thousands of genetic diseases are now known', neglect to mention that the 'scientific literature' supporting their claim is infinitely more 'anecdotal' than the despised 'anecdotal' support for the various unofficial remedies that are so offensive to the medical establishment. ... Sanity itself requires that we do not confuse our wishes, methods, assumptions and ideas, with the world that we are trying to understand. **If our method determines our conclusions, we are closer to theology than to science, and that is how many 'scientists' prefer it** (my emphasis)."

When will medicine learn that describing a disease in terms of a specific cause, is as erroneous as describing the glorious voice of a great singer as simply a matter of vibrating vocal chords. The majority of diseases today are caused by what humankind has done to their environment. This cannot be questioned any longer, the proof is irrefutable. What is an even greater sadness, is that the efforts designed to correct these diseases usually adds to the suffering and a quicker demise.

Only through the efforts of the people can the right to choose one's own path to better health be won. Let the information be available. All governments should let the public know that a particular therapy has not met the so-called scientific proof of today and allow them to make the choice, especially when the alternative substance has been in use for many years (often thousands) without any evidence of toxicity or deaths and, in fact, is usually classified as a food. To force individuals to except the failure of medical therapy as their only choice is unconscionable. To promulgate the medical myth, that theirs is the only solution, is depraved and corrupt.

****

AN IMPORTANT REMINDER

The National Cancer Institute tells us that 65% to 75% of all cancers can be avoided with 2 or more lifestyle changes. I firmly believe that if all the precautions indicated in this book were initiated more than 95% of all cancers could be prevented. It would follow logically that many preventive techniques are obviously effective therapeutically.

Chapter 19

A Helping Hand

PROFESSIONAL RESOURCES

COMPREHENSIVE PRACTITIONERS OF COMPLEMENTARY AND ALTERNATIVE THERAPIES, CHELATION AND OTHER COMPLEMENTARY TECHNIQUES

THE UNITED STATES

ALABAMA

Birmingham

P. Gus J. Prosch Jr. MD, (205) 823-6180

ALASKA

Anchorage

F. Rusell Manuel, MD (907) 562-7070

Robert Rowen,MD (907) 344-7775

Soldotna

Paul G. Isaak, MD (907) 262-9341

Wasilla Robert E. Martin, MD (907) 376-5284

ARIZONA

Glendale

Lloyd D. Armold, DO (602) 939-8916

Mesa

William W. Halcomb, DO (602) 832-3014

Parker

S. W. Meyer, DO (602) 669-8911

Pheonix

Terry S. Friedmann MD (602) 381-0800

Stanley R. Olsztyn, MD (602) 954-0811

Prescott

Gordon H. Josephs, DO (602) 778-6169

Scottsdale

Gordon H. Josephs, DO (602) 998-9232

Tempe

Garry Gordon, MD (602) 838-2079

ARKANSAS

Hot Springs

William Wright, MD (501) 624-3312

Leslie

Melissa Taliaferro, MD (501) 447-2599

Little Rock

Norbert J. Becquet, MD (501) 375-4419

John L. Gustavus, MD (501) 758-9350

Springdale

Doty Murphy Ill. MD (501) 756-3251

CALIFORNIA

Albany

Ross B. Gordon, MD (510) 526-3232

Auburn

Zane Kime, MD, (916) 823-3421

Bakersfield

Ralph G. Seibly, MD (805) 873-1000

Campbell

Carol A Shamlin, MD (408) 378-7970

Chico

Eva Jalkotzy, MD (916) 893-3080

Concord

John P. Toth, Gossypol MD (510) 682-5660

Corte Madera

Michael Rosenbaum,MD (415) 927-9450

Covina

James Privitera, MD, (818) 966-1618

Daly City

Charles K. Dahlgren, MD (415) 756-2900

El Cajon

William J. Saccoman, MD (619) 440-3838

Encino

A. Leonard Klepp, MD, (818) 981-5511

Fresno

David J. Edwards, MD (209) 251-5066

Grand Terrace

Bruce Halstead, MD, (714) 783-2773

Hollywood

James J. Julian, MD (213) 467-5555

Joan Priestley, MD, (213) 957-4217

Huntington Beach
>Joan M. Resk, DO, (714) 842-5591

Lake Forest
>David A. Steenblock, DO (714) 770-9616

Laytonville
>Eugene D. Finkle, MD (707) 984-6151

Long Beach
>H. Richard Casdorph, MD (310) 597-8716

Los Altos
>Robert F. Cathcart Ill. MD (415) 949-2822

>Claude Marquette, MD (415) 964-6700

Los Angeles
>Laszio Belenyessy, MD, (213) 822-4614

>M. Jahangiri, MD, (213) 587-3218

Monterey
>Lon B. Work, MD, (408) 655-0215

Newport Beach
>Julian Whitaker,MD (714) 851-1550

North Hollywood
>David C. Freeman, MD (818) 985-1103

Oxnard
>Mohamed Moharram, MD, (805) 483-2355

Palm Desert
>David H. Tang, MD,

Palm Springs
>Sean Degnan, MD, (619) 320-4292

Porterville
John B. Park, MD, (209) 781-6224

Rancho Mirage
Charles Farinella, MD, (619) 324-0734

Redding
Bessie J. Tillman, MD, (916) 246-3022

Reseda
Ilona Abraham, MD, (818) 345-8721

Sacramento
Michael Kwiker, DO, (916) 489-4400

San Diego
Lawrence Taylor, MD, (619) 296-2952

San Francisco
Richard A. Kunin, MD, (415) 346-2500

Russell A. Lemesh, MD, (415) 731-5907 281

Paul Lynn, MD, (415) 566-1000

Gary S. Ross, MD, (41) 398-0555

San Leandro
Steven H. Gee, MD, (510) 483-5881

San Rafael
Ross B. Gordon, MD, (41) 499-9377

San Marcos
William C. Kubitschek, DO, (619) 744-6991

Santa Ana
Ana Ronald Wempen, MD, (714) 546-4325

Santa Barbara

H. J. Hoegerman,MD, (805) 963-1824

Mohamed Moharam, MD, (805) 965-5229

Santa Maria

Donald E. Reiner, MD, (805) 925-0961

Santa Monica

Michael Rosenbaum,MD, (310) 453-4424

Murray Susser, MD, (310) 453-4424

Santa Rosa

Terri Su, MD, (707) 571-7560

Seal Beach

Allen Green, MD, (310) 493-4526

Smith River

JoAnn Hoffer, MD, (707) 487-3405 282

James D. Schuler, MD, (707) 487-3405

Stanton

William J. Goldwag, MD, (714) 827-5180

Studio City

Charles E. Law Jr. MD, (818) 761-1661

Torrance

Anita Millen, MD, (310) 320-1132

Van Nuys

Frank Mosler, MD, (818) 785-7425

Walnut Creek

Alan Shifman Charles,MD, (510) 937-3331

Peter H. C. Mutke, MD, (510) 933-2405

COLORADO

Colorado Springs
>Sandra Denton, MD, (719) 548-1600

>James R. Fish, MD, (719) 471-2273

>George Juetersonke, DO, (719) 528-1960

Englewood
>John H. Altshuler, MD, (303) 740-7771

Grand Junction
>William L. Reed, MD., (303) 241-3631

CONNECTICUT

Torrington
>Jerrold N. Finnie, MD, (203) 489-8977

DISTRICT OF COLUMBIA

Washington
>Paul Beals, MD, (202) 332-0370

>George H. Mitchell, MD, (202) 265-4111

FORIDA

Boca Raton
>Leonard Haimes, MD, (407) 994-3868

>Narinder Singh Parhar, MD, (407) 479-3200

Bradenton
>Eteri Meinkov, MD, (813) 748-7943

Fort Lauderdale
>Bruce Dooley, MD, (305) 527-9355

Fort Myers
>Gary L. Pynckel, DO., (813) 278-3377

Hollywood

Herbert Pardell, DO, (305) 989-5558

Homosassa

Carolos F. Gonzalez, MD, (904) 382-282

Jupiter

Neil Ahner, MD, (407) 744-0077

Lakeland

Harold Robinson, MD, (813) 646-5088

Lauderhill

Herbert R. Slavin, MD, (305) 748-4991

Maitland

Joya Lynn Schoen, MD, (407) 644-29

Miami

Stanley J. Cannon, MD, (305) 279-3020

Joseph G. Godorov, DO, (305) 595-0671

Bernard J. Letourneau, DO, (305) 666-9933

North Lauderdale

Narinder Singh Parhar, MD, (305) 978-6604

North Miami Beach

Martin Dayton, DO, (305) 931-8484

Ocala

George Graves, DO, (904)236-2525 or
(904) 732-3633

Orange City

Travis L. Herring, MD, (904) 775-0525

Palm Bay

Neil Ahner, MD, (407)729-8581

Pompano Beach
>Dan C. Roehm, MD, (305) 977-3700

Port Canaveral
>James Parsons, MD., (407) 784-2102

Sarasota
>Joseph Ossorio, MD, (813) 921-6338

St. Petersburg
>Ray Wunderlich, Jr. MD, (813) 822-3612

Tampa
>Donald J. Carrow, MD, (813) 832-3220

>Eugene H. Lee, MD, (813) 251-3089

Venice
>Thomas McNaughton, MD, (813) 484-2167

Wauchula
>Alfred S. Massam, MD, (813) 773-6668

Winter Park
>James M. Parsons, MD, (407) 628-3399

>Robert R. Rogers, MD, (407) 679-2811

GEORGIA

Atlanta
>David Epstein, DO, (404) 525-7333

>Milton Fried, MD, (404) 451-4857

>Bernard Mlaver, MD, (404) 39500

Camilla
>Oliver M. Gunter, MD, (912) 336-7343

Decatur

    Naima ABD Elghany, MD, (404) 639-3385

Norcross

    Stephen Edelson, MD, (404) 729-8359

Waner Robins

    Terril J. Schneider, MD, (912) 929-1027

HAWAII

Kailua-Kona

    Clifton Arrington, MD, (808) 322-9400

IDAHO

Coeur d'Alene

    Charles T. McGee, MD, (208) 664-1478

Nampa

    John O. Boxall, MD, (208) 466-3517

    Stephen Thornburgh, DO, (208) 466-3517

Sandpoint

    K. Peter McCallum MD, (208) 263-5456

ILLINOIS

Arlington Heights

    Terrill K. Haws, DO, (708) 577-9451

    William J. Mauer, DO, (800) 255-7030

Aurora

    Thomas Hesselink, MD, (708) 844-0011

Belvidere

    M. Paul Dommers, MD, (815) 544-3112 287

Chicago

    Razvan Rentea MD, (312) 549-0101

Geneva

Richard E. Hrdlicka,MD, (708) 232-1900

Glen Ellyn

Robert S. Waters, MD, (708) 790-8100

Metamora

Stephen K. Elsasser, DO, (309) 367-2321

Moline

Tery W. Love, DO, (309) 764-2900

Oak Park

Paul J. Dunn, MD, (708) 383-3800

Ottawa

Terry W. Love, DO, (815) 434-1977

Woodstock

John R.Tambone, MD, (815) 338-2345

Zion Peter Senatore, DO, (708) 872-8722

INDIANA

Clarksville

George Wolverton, MD, (812) 282-4309

Evansville

Harold T. Sparks, DO, (812) 479-8228

Highland

Cal Streeter, DO, (219) 924-240

Indianapolis

David A. Darbro, MD, (317) 787-7221 288

Mooresville

Norman E. Whitney, DO, (317) 831-3352

South Bend

David E. Turfler, DO, (219) 233-3840

Valparaiso

Myrna D. Trowbridge, DO, (219) 462-3377

IOWA

Des Moines

Beverly Rosenfeld, DO, (515) 276-0061

Sioux City

Horst G. Blume, MD, (712) 252-4386

KANSAS

Andover

Stevens B. Acker, MD, (316) 733-4494

Garden City

Terry Hunsberger, DO, (316) 275-7128

Hays

Roy N. Neil, MD, (913) 628-8341

Kansas City

John Gamble Jr. DO, (913) 321-1140

KENTUCKY

Bowling Green

John C Tapp, MD, (502) 781-1483

Louisville

Kirk Morgan, MD, (502) 228-0156

Nicholasville

Walt Stoll, MD, (606) 233-4273

Somerset

Stephen S. Kiteck, MD, (606) 678-5137

LOUISIANA

Chalmette

Jaroj T. Tampira, MD, (504) 277-8991

Manderville

Roy M. Montalbano, MD, (504) 626-1985

Natchitoches

Phillip Mitchell, MD, (318) 357-1571 or
(800) 562-6574

Newellton

Joseph R. Whitaker, MD, (318) 467-5131

New Iberia

Adonis J. Domingue,MD, (318) 365-2196

New Orleans

James P. Carter, MD, (504) 588-5136

Shreveport

R. Denman Crow, MD, (318) 221-1569

MAINE

Van Buren

Joseph Cyr, MD, (207) 868-5273

MARYLAND

Laurel

Paul V. Beals, MD, (301) 490-9911 290

Pikesville

Alan R. Gaby, MD, (410) 486-5656a

Rockville

Harold Goodman, DO, (301) 881-5229

MASSACHUSETS

Barnstable

Michael Jansen, MD, (508) 362-4343

Cambridge

Michael Jansen, MD, (617) 661-6225

Hanover

Richard Cohen, MD, (617) 829-9281

Lowell

Svetlana Kaufman, MD, (508) 453-5181

Newton

Carol Englender, MD, (617) 965-7770

West Boylston

N. Thomas La Cava, MD, (508) 854-1380

Williamstown

Ross S. McConnell, MD, (413) 663-3701

MICHIGAN

Atlanta

Leo Modzinski DO, MD, (517) 785-4254

Bay City

Doyle B. Hill, DO, (517) 686-5200

Farmington Hills

Paul A. Parente, DO, (313) 626-7544 291

Albert J.Scarchilli, DO, (313) 626-7544

Flint

William M. Bernard, DO, (313) 733-3140

Kenneth Ganapini, DO, (313) 733-3140

Grand Rapids

Grant Born, DO, (616) 455-3550

Linden

Marvin D. Penwell, DO, (313) 735-7809

Pontiac
Vahagn Agbabian, DO, (313) 334-2424

St. Clair Shores
Richard E. Tapert, DO, (313) 779-5700

Williamston
Seldon Nelson, DO, (517) 349-248

MINNESOTA
Minneapolis
Michael Dole, MD, (612) 593-9458

Jean R. Eckerly, MD, (612) 593-9458

Tyler
Keith J. Carlson, MD, (507) 247-5921

MISSISSIPPI
Coldwater
Pravinchandra Patel, MD, (601) 622-7011

Columbus
James H. Sams, MD, (601) 327-8701

Ocean Springs
James H. Waddell, MD, (601) 875-5505

Shelby
Robert Hollingsworth, MD, (601) 398-5106

MISSOURI
Festus
John T. Schwent, DO, (314) 937-8688

Florissant
Tipu Sultan,MD, (314) 921-7100

Independence
Lawrence Dorman, DO, (816) 358-2712

James E. Swann, DO, (816) 833-3366

Kansas City

Edward W. McDonagh, DO, (816) 453-5940

James Rowland, DO, (816) 361-4077

Charles J. Rudolph, DO, (816) 453-5940

Springfield

William C. Sunderwirth, DO, (417) 869-6260

St. Louis

Harvey Walker Jr. MD, (314) 721-7227

Stockton

William C. Sunderwirth, DO, (417) 276-3221

Sullivan

Ronald H. Scott, DO, (314) 468-4932

Union

Clinton C. Hayes, DO, (314) 583-8911

NEBRASKA

Omaha

Eugene C. Oliveto, MD, (402) 392-0233

Ord

Otis W. Miller, MD, (308) 728-3251

NEVADA

Incline Village

W. Douglas Brodie,MD, (702) 83207001

Las Vegas

Ji-Zhou (Joseph) Kang, MD, (702) 798-2992

Robert D. Milne, MD, (702) 385-1999

Terry Pfau, DO, (702) 385-1999

Robert Vance, DO, (702) 385-7771

Reno

David A. Edwards, MD, (702) 827-1444

Michael L. Gerber, MD, (702) 826-1900

Donald E. Soli, MD, (702) 786-7101 294

Yiwen Y. Tang, MD, (702) 826-9500

NEW JERSEY

Cherry Hill

Allan Magaziner, DO, (609) 424-8222

Denville

Majid Ali, MD, (201) 586-4111

Edison

C. Y. Lee, MD, (908) 738-9220

Ralph Lev, MD, (908) 738-9220

Richard B. Menashe, DO, (908) 906-8866

Elizabethtown

Gennaro Locurcio, MD, (908) 31-1333

Ortley Beach

Charles Harris, MD, (908) 793-6464

Ridgewood

Constance Alfano, MD, (201) 444-4622

Skillman

Eric Braverman, MD, (609) 921-1842

West Orange

    Faina Muntis, MD, (201) 736-3743

NEW MEXICO

Alburquerque

    Ralph J. Luciani, DO, (505) 888-5995 295

    Gerald Parker, DO, (505) 884-3506

    John T. Taylor, DO, (505) 884-3506

Roswell

    Annette Stoesser, MD, (505) 623-2444

NEW YORK

Bronx

    Richard Izquierdo, MD, (212) 589-4541

Brooklyn

    Gennaro Locurcio, MD, (718) 336-2291

    Tsilia Sorina, MD, (718) 375-2600

    Michael Teplitsky, MD, (718) 769-0997

    Pavel Yutsis, MD, (718) 259-2122

East Meadow

    Christopher Calapai, DO, (516) 794-0404

Falconer

    Reino Hill, MD, (716) 665-3505

Huntington

    Serafina Corsello, MD, (516) 271-0222

Lawrence

    Mitchell Kurk, MD, (516) 239-5540

Massena

Bob Snider, MD, (315) 764-7328

New York

Robert C. Atkins, MD, (212) 758-2110

Serafina Corsello, MD, (212) 399-0222

Ronald Hoffman, MD, (212) 779-1744

Warren M. Levin, MD, (212) 696-1900

Niagara Falls

Paul Cutler, MD, (716) 284-5140

Orangeburg

Neil L.Block, MD, (914) 359-3300

Plattsburgh

Driss Hassam, MD, (518) 561-2023

Rhinebeck

Kenneth A. Bock,MD, (914) 876-7082

Suffern

Michael B. Schachter, MD, (914) 368-4700

Watervliet

Rodolfo T. Sy, MD, (518) 273-1325

Westbury

Savely Yurkovsky, MD, (516) 333-2929

NORTH CAROLINA

Aberdeen

Keith E. Johnson, MD, (919) 281-5122 297

Leicester

John L. Laird, MD, (704) 876-1617

Statesville

John L. Laird, MD, (704) 876-1617
(800) 445-4762

NORTH DAKOTA

Grand Forks

Richard H. Leigh, MD, (701) 775-5527

Minot

Brian E. Briggs, MD, (701) 838-6011

OHIO

Akron

Josephine Aronica, MD, (216) 867-7361

Francis J. Waickman, MD, (216) 867-3767

Bluffton L. Terry Chappell, MD, (419) 358-4627

Canton

Jack E. Slingluff DO, (216) 494-8641

Cincinnati

Ted Cole, DO, (513) 779-0300

Cleveland

John M. Baron, DO, (216) 642-0082

James P. Frackelton, MD, (216) 835-0104

Derrick Lonsdale, MD, (216) 835-0104

Douglas Weeks, MD, (216) 835-0104

Columbus

Robert R. Hershner, DO, (614) 253-8733

William D. Mitchell, DO, (614) 761-0555

Dayton

David D. Goldberg, DO, (513) 277-1722

Lancaster

Richard Sielski, MD, (614) 653-0017

Paulding

Don K. Snyder, MD, (419) 399-2045

Youngstown

James Ventresco Jr., DO, (216) 792-2349

OKLAHOMA

Jenks

Leon Anderson, DO, (918) 299-5039

Oklahoma City

Charles H. Farr, MD, (405) 632-8868

Charles D. Taylor, MD, (405) 525-7751

OREGON

Ashland

Ronald L. Peters, MD, (503) 482-7007

Eugene

John Gambee, MD, (503) 686-2536

Grants Pass

James Fitzsimmons Jr., MD, (503) 474-2166

Salem

Terence Howe Young, MD, (503) 371-1558

PENNSYLVANIA

Allentown

Robert H. Schmidt, DO, (215) 437-1959

D. Erik Von Kiel, DO, (215) 776-7639

Bangor

Francis J. Cinelli, DO, (215) 588-4502

Bedford

Bill Illingworth, DO, (814) 623-8414

Bethlehem

Sally Ann Rex, DO, (215) 866-0900

Ellizabethtown

Dennis L. Gilbert, DO, (717) 367-134

Fountainville

Harold H. Byer, MD, (215) 348-0443

Greensburg

R. A. Miranda, MD, (412) 838-7632

Hazleton

Arthur L. Koch, DO, (717) 455-4747

Indiana

Chandrika Sinha, MD, (412) 349-1414 300

Macungie

D. Erik Von Kiel, DO, (215) 967-5503

Mertztown

Conrad G. Maulfair Jr, DO., (215) 682-2104

Mt. Pleasant

Mamduh El-Attrache, MD, (412) 547-3576

North Versailles

Mamduh El-Attrache, MD, (412) 673-3900

Philadelphia

Frederick Burton, MD, (215) 844-4660

Jose Castillo, MD, (215) 567-5845,46,47

Mura Galperin, MD, (21) 677-2337

P. Jayalakshmi, MD, (215) 473-4226

K. R. Sampathachar, MD, (215) 473-4226

Lance Wright, MD, (21) 387-1200

Quakertown

Harold Buttram, MD, (215) 536-1890

Somerset Paul Peirsel, MD, (814) 443-2521

SOUTH CAROLINA

Columbia

Theodore C. Rozema, MD, (803) 796-1702
(800) 992-8350

Landrum

Theodore C.Rozema, MD, (803) 457-4141
(800) 992-8350

TENNESSE

Morristown

Donald Thompson, MD, (615) 581-6367

Nashville

Stephen L. Reisman, MD, (615) 383-9030

TEXAS

Alamo

Herbert Carr, DO, (512) 787-6668

Abilene

William Irby Fox, MD, (915) 672-7863

Amarillo

Gerald Parker, DO, (806) 355-8263

John T. Taylor DO, (806) 355-8263

Austin

Vladimir Rizov, MD, (512) 451-8149

Dallas

Brij Myer, MD, (214) 248-2488

Michael G. Samuels, DO, (214) 991-3977

J. Robert Winslow, DO, (214) 241-4614

J. Robert Winslow, DO, (214) 243-7711

El Paso

Edward J. Etti, MD, (915) 566-9361

Francisco Soto, MD, (915) 534-0272

Houston

Robert Battle, MD, (713) 932-0552

Jerome L. Borochoff, MD, (713) 461-7517

Luis E. Guerrero, MD, (713) 789-0133

Humble

John P. Trowbridge, MD, (713) 540-39

Kirbyville John L. Sessions, DO, (409) 423-2166

La Porte

Ronald M. Davis, MD, (713) 470-2930

Pecos

Ricardo Tan, MD, (915) 445-9090

Plano

Linda Martin, DO, (214) 985-1377

San Antonio

Ron Stogryn, MD, (512) 366-3637 303

Wichita Falls

Thomas R. Humphrey, MD, (817) 766-4329

UTAH

Provo

Dennis Harper, DO, (801) 373-8500

D. Remington, MD, (801) 373-8500

VIRGINIA

Annandale

Sohini Patel, MD, (703) 941-3606

Hinton

Harold Huffman, MD, (703) 867-5242

Midlothian

Peter C. Gent, DO, (804) 744-3551

Norfolk

Vincent Speckhart, MD, (804) 622-0014

Trout

Dale Elmer M. Cranton, MD, (703) 677- 3631

WASHINGTON

Bellevue

David Buscher, MD, (206) 453-0288

Bellingham

Robert Kimmel, MD, (206) 734-3250

Kent

Jonathan Wright, MD, (206) 631-892 304

Kirkland

Jonathan Collin, MD, (206) 820-0547

Port Townsend

Jonathan Collin, MD, (206) 385-4555

Seattle

Michael G. Vesselago, MD, (206) 367-0760

Spokane

Burton B. Hart, DO, (509) 927-9922

Vancouver

Richard P. Huemer, MD, (206) 253-4445

Yakima

Murray L. Black, DO, (509) 966-1780

Yelm

Elmer M. Cranton, MD, (206) 894-3548

WEST VIRGINIA

Beckley

Purencio Corro, MD, (304) 252-0775

Michael Kostenko, DO, (304) 0591

Charleston

Steve M. Zekan, MD, (304) 343-7559

WISCONSIN

Green Bay

Eleazar M. Kadie, MD, (414) 468-9442

Lake Geneva

Rathna Alwa, MD, (414) 248-1430 305

Milwaukee

William J. Faber, DO, (414) 467-7680

Thomas Hesselink, MD, (414) 259-1350

Jerry N. Yee, DO, (414) 258-6282

Wisconsin Dells

Robert S. Waters, MD, (608) 254-7178

INTERNATIONAL

THERE ARE MANY MORE PRACTITIONERS THAN THOSE LISTED HERE, WHO CAN PROVIDE THE SERVICES YOU REQUIRE. THESE PRACTITIONERS CAN ALWAYS REFER YOU TO ONE OF THEIR COLLEAGUES WHOSE OFFICES MAY BE MORE ACCESSIBLE OR OFFER A THERAPY THAT THEY DON'T. THEY VERY OFTEN WILL DIRECT YOU TO A PROFESSIONAL ORGANIZATION IN YOUR COUNTRY WHICH HAS A COMPLETE LISTING. I AM LISTING INDIVIDUALS THAT I HAVE PERSONALLY MET OR WHOSE CREDENTIALS SPEAK WELL FOR THEM.

AUSTRALIA

Victoria

Donvale R. B. Allen, MD, 011-43-247-388

NEW SOUTH WALES

Artarmon

Heather M. Bassett, MD, (043) 24-7388

Beecroft

Heather M. Bassett, MD, (043) 24-7388
(043) 23-6785

Chatswood

Tony Goh, MD, 411-5011

Gosford

Heather M. Bassett, MD, (043) 24 7388

Mosman

Emmanuel Varipatis, MD, 2-0604133 307

BAHAMAS

Nassau

Michael Ingraham, MD, (809) 323-3530

BELGIUM

Antwerpen

Rudy Proesmans, MD, 011-32-3-2250313

Ghent

Michel De Meyer, MD, 091-22-33-42

Tienen

Marc Verheyen, MD, 011-32-1681 8393

BRAZIL

Curitiba

Oslim Malina, MD, 011-41-2524395

Florianopolis

Jose P. Figueredo, 011-482-22-4960

Osorio-RS

Jose Valdai de Souza, MD, 011-55-51-6641269

Pelotas-RS

Antonio C. Fernandes, MD, 011-55-53-2224699

Porto Alegre

Moyses Hodara, MD, 011-55-51-2243557

Sao Paulo

Guilherme Deucher, MD, 011-55-11-5719100

Wagner Fiori, MD, 011-55-11-2112019

Fernando L. Flaquer, MD, 011-55-2112019

Carlos Eduardo Leite, MD, 011-55-11-4693899

Wilson Rondo, MD, 011-55-11-820-4990

Sergio Vaisman, MD, 011-55-11-2108210

CANADA

ALBERTA

Calgary

Louis Grondin, MD, (403)245-8008

J. Soriano-Grondin, MD, (403) 245-8008.

Edmonton

Tris Trethart, MD, (403) 433-7401

K. B. Wiancko, MD, (403) 483-2703

BRITISH COLUMBIA

Errington

George Barber, MD, (604) 248-8956

Kelowna

Alex A. Neil, MD, (604) 765-2145

Vancouver

Saul Pilar, MD, (604) 739-8858

Donald W. Stewart , MD, (604) 736-1105

Zigurts Strauts, MD, (604) 736-1105

MANITOBA

Winnepeg

Howard N. Reed, MD, (204) 957-1900

ONTARIO

Blythe

Richard W. Street, MD, (519) 523-4433

Smiths Falls

Clare Minielly, MD, (613) 283-7703

Willowdale

Paul Cutler, MD, (416) 733-3151

COSTA RICA

San Jose

Fabio Solano, MD, (506) 39-00-22

DENMARK

Aabyjoej

Kurt Christensen, MD, 06-126141

Copenhagen

Sven Feddersen, MD, 945-31-584114

Humlebaek

Joergen Rugaard, MD, 42 19 09 09 310

Lyngby

Claus Hanckce, MD, 45 42 88 09 00

Skodsborg

Bo Moglevang, MD, 011-4542803200

Vejle

Knut T. Flytlie, MD, 011-4575820346

Viby

Bruce P. Kyle, MD, 86-293550

DOMINICAN REPUBLIC

Santo Domingo

Antonio Pannocchia, MD, 565-3259

EGYPT

Cairo

Elham G. Behery, MD, 011-202-3484517

ENGLAND

Kent

F. Schellander, MD, 011-44-892-543536

Lancashire

Tarsem Lai Garg, MD, 0942-676617

London

Tarsem Lai Garg, MD, 071-486-1095 or
071-486-3812

West Sussex

Semi Khanna, MD, 011-44-342-324984

FRANCE

Paris

Bruno Crussol, MD, 011-33-1 47551919

Paul Musarella, MD, 011-33-1-45621938

GERMANY

Bad Fussing

Karl Heinz Caspers, MD, 011-49-8531-21001 or
011-49-8531-21004

Bad Steben

Helmut Keller, MD 011-49-9288-5166

Bremerhaven

Reiner W. Theis, MD, 0471-52066

Langenhagen

Hans A. Nieper, 49-511-348-0808

Rottach-Egern

Claus Martin, MD, 011-49-8022-6415

Werne

Jens-Ruediger Collatz, MD, 02389-3883

INDONESIA

Bandung

Benj. Widjajakusuma, MD, 011-62-22-615277

Jakarta

Maimunah Affandi, MD, 011-62-21-716927

Laurentius Dermawan, MD, 011-62-21-7697525

Yahya Kisyanto, MD, 011-62-21-334636 312

Hendra Setiady, MD, 011-62-21-4713880

Dien G. H. Tan, MD, 011-62-21-7203476

Rini J. Utama, MD, 011-62-21-680-343

Semarang

Benny Purwanto, MD, 011-62-24-516-275

ITALY
Palermo

Michele Ballo, MD, 91-580301

KOREA
Seoul

J. K. Hyun, MD, 011-82-2-514-7832

MALAYSIA
Melaka

Mohamed S. A. Ishak, MD, 06-235878 or
06-239396

MEXICO
Chihuahua

H. Berlanga Reyes, MD, (95) 141-3-92-71 or
(95) 141-3-92-75

Guadelajara, Jalisco

Eleazar A. Carrasco, MD, 25-16-55

F. Navares Merino, MD, (36) 16-88-70

Juarez, Chih.

H. Berlanga, Reyes, MD, 13-80-23

Francisco Soto, MD, 52-16-162-601

Matamoros, Tamp.
Frank Morales Sr., MD, 3-31-07

Tijuana

Jose A. Calzada, MD, 011-52-66-342233

Francisco Rique, MD, (706) 681-3171

Rodrigo Rodriguez, MD, (706) 681-3171

Roberto Tapia, MD, (706) 681-3171

Torreon, Coahuila
Carlos Lopez Moreno, MD, 011-52-17-138140

NETHERLANDS

Etten-Leur

Peter Zeegers, MD, 011-31-1608-17127

Haarlem

Eduard Schweden, MD, 011-31-23-328833

Leende

P. van der Schaar, MD, 011-31-4959-2232

Marc Verheyen, MD, 011-31-4959-2232

Loenersloot

A. Verbon, MD 011-31-2949-1289

Maastricht

Rob van Zandvoort, MD, 011-31-4362-3474

Oudenbosch

E. T. Oei, MD, 011-31-1652-17455

Rotterdam

Robert T. J. K. Trossel, MD,
01131 10 4126362/4147633

Velp J. H. Leenders, MD, 31-085-642742

NETHERLANDS-ANTILLES
Aruba

Adhemar E. Hart, MD, 011-297-8-27263

St. Maarten

Sharon Ruth Brandon, MD, 011-5995-53097

Robert T. H. K. Trossel, MD, 011-5995-53097

NEW ZEALAND
Auckland

Maurice B. Archer, DO, 011-64-9-524-7743, 45 or 48

R. H. Bundeliu, MD, 011-64-9-2746701 315

Raymond Ramirez, MD, (09) 872-200.

Christchurch

Robert Blackmore, MD, (03) 853-015

Masterton

T. J. Baily Gibson, MD, (059) 81-250

Napier

Tony Edwards, MD, (070) 354-696

Oxford, N. Canterbury
Ted Walford, MD, (075) 86-808

Tauranga

Michael E. Godfrey, MD, (075) 782-362

NORWAY
Svinndal

Arild Abrahamsen, MD, 011-9-286065

PANAMA

Panama City

Frank Ferro, MD, 011-507-27-4733, ext. 190

PHILIPPINES

Manila

Rosa M. Ami Belli, MD, 50-03-23

Leonides Lerma, MD, 57-59-11

Corazon

Macawili-Yu, MD, 50-03-23

Remedios L. Reynoso, MD, 50--3-23

PUERTO RICO

Guayanilla, P.R.

Miguel A. Santos, MD, (809) 835-0649

Santurce

Pedro Zayas,, MD, (809) 727-1105

SPAIN

Madrid

Dirk van Lith, MD, c/o Prof. Joaquin Prieto.

SWITZERLAND

Geneva

Robert Tissot, MD, (22) 498875

Montreux

Claude Rossel, MD, 21-6351-01

Netstal (Glarus)

Walter Blumer, MD, 058-61-28-46

TAIWAN (R.O.C.)

Taipei

Paul Lin, MD, (02) 507-2222 (Teipei) Ext. 1003

Yeh-Sung Lin, MD, 886-2-507-8349 317

VENEZUELA
Puerto La Cruz

Rosella Mazzuka, MD, 011-58-81-691272

WEST INDIES

JAMAICA
Montego Bay
H. Marco Brown, MD, 011-809-952-3454

****

ORIENTAL MEDICINE, NATUROPATHIC MEDICINE and NUTRITION
Bastyr College, Natural Health Sciences, 144 N.E. 54th, Seattle, WA 98105. Phone: (206) 523-9585.

AYURVEDIC PRACTITIONERS:
Scott Gerson, MD, Ayurvedic Medicine of New York, 13 West 9th St., New York, NY, Phone: (212) 505-8971.

Karta Purkh Khalsa, Health Ceter, 1305 Northeast 45th St., Suite 205, Seattle, WA Phone: (206) 547-2007. Fax: (206) 547-4240.

PRACTITIONERS OF TRADITIONAL CHINESE MEDICINE
Betances Health Unit, 281 East Broadway, New York, NY 10002. Phone: (212) 227-8843.

Holistically-oriented clinic Dr. Daniel Hsu c/o Oriental Healing Arts Institute, 1945 Palo Verde Ave., Suite 208, Long Beach, CA 90815. Phone: (310) 431-3544. Treating Cancer with Chineses Herbs ($12.95) and other materials. Ask for catalog.

Miki Shima, OMD, Lic.Ac. (Dr. of Oriental Medicine, Licensed Acupunturist) 21 Tamal Vista Boulevard, Suite 110, Corte

Madera, CA 94925. Phone: (415) 924-2910. Fax: (415) 924-5072.

Dr. Binyan Sun, 463 James Road, Palo Alto, CA 94306. Phone: (415) 858-0320. Chinese speaking patients only: (415) 858-2520.

PRODUCT RESOURCES

DISCOUNT AND MAIL ORDER SOURCE FOR MOST ITEMS

Life Extension Foundation, 2490 Griffin Road, Fort Lauderdale, FL 33312 Phone: 800 841-5433, (305) 966-4886.

Donigan Nutrition Center, 2621 North Federal Highway Boca Raton, FL 33431. Phone: (407) 395-5521.

Check your local directories for possible discount stores and chains.

Acidophilus

Ecological Formulas, 1061-B Shary Circle, Concord, CA 94518. Phone: 800 888-4585. (510) 827-2636 Fax (510) 676-9231.

Klaire Laboratories, Inc., PO Box 618, Carsbad, CA 92008/0010. Phone: (619) 744-9680. or 4 Museum St. York, YO1 2ES, England. Phone: 0904-52378.

Natren, 10935 Camarillo Street, North Hollywood, CA 91602. Phone: (800) 992-3233 or (800) 992-9393.

GY&N Nutrient Pharmacology P.O. Box 2252, Carlsbad, CA 92018 (619) 434-6360, 800 445-2122, Fax (619) 434-0816.

Aloe products

Allergy Research Group, PO Box 489/400 Preda Street, San Lenadro, CA 94577-0489. Phone: (415) 639-4572.

Klabin Marketing, 115 Central Park West, New York, NY 10023. Phone: 800 933-9440.

Amino acids

Allergy Research Group, PO Box 489/400 Preda Street, San Lenadro, CA 94577-0489. Phone: (415) 639-4572 or 800 545-9960.

Ecological Formulas, 1061-B Shary Circle, Concord, CA 94518. Phone: 800 888-4585. (510) 827-2636 Fax (510) 676-9231.

Jo Mar Laboratories, 251 East Hacienda Avenue, Campbell CA 95008. Phone 800 538-4545 or 800 847-8855.

GY&N Nutrient Pharmacology P.O. Box 2252, Carlsbad, CA 92018 (619) 434-6360, 800 445-2122, Fax (619) 434-0816.

Amygdalin (B-17), Laetrile

There are only two sources that I would trust in order to obtain bioactive Amygdalin for intravenous administration.

Andrew McNaughton c/o The McNaughton Foundation, 416 W. San Isidro Blvd., Suite L-666, San Ysidro, CA 92173.

C.P.W. Rahlstedt, Box 73 0527, D-W-2000 Hamburg, Germany.

Anticoagulants

Leo R. Zacharski, MD. Phone: (802) 296-5149.

Antioxidants

Ecological Formulas, 1061-B Shary Circle, Concord, CA 94518. Phone: 800 888-4585. (510) 827-2636 Fax (510) 676-9231.

Allergy Research Group, PO Box 489/400 Preda Street, San Lenadro, CA 94577-0489. Phone: (415) 639-4572.

Miller Pharmacal Group 4563 Prime Parkway Dr. P.O. Box 1297 Mc Henry, Illinois, 60050-1297. Phone: 800 323-2935.

GY&N Nutrient Pharmacology P.O. Box 2252, Carlsbad, CA 92018 (619) 434-6360, 800 445-2122, Fax (619) 434-0816.

Antineoplastons
Burzynski Research Institute, Outpatient Department, 6221 Corporate Drive, Houston, Texas. Phone: (713) 777-8233.

Arginine (see Amino Acids)
Allergy Research Group, PO Box 489/400 Preda Street, San Lenadro, CA 94577-0489. Phone: (415) 639-4572.

Ecological Formulas, 1061-B Shary Circle, Concord, CA 94518. Phone: 800 888-4585. (510) 827-2636 Fax (510) 676-9231.

GY&N Nutrient Pharmacology P.O. Box 2252, Carlsbad, CA 92018 (619) 434-6360, 800 445-2122, Fax (619) 434-0816.

Jo Mar Laboratories, 251 East Hacienda Avenue, Campbell, CA 95008. Phone: 800 538-4545.

Aristolochia Acid (KC2)
C.P.W. Rahlstedt P.O. Box 73 05 27 D-W-2000 Hamburg 73 Germany.

Astragalus (see Herbs)
Ecological Formulas, 1061-B Shary Circle, Concord, CA 94518. Phone: 800 888-4585. (510) 827-2636 Fax (510) 676-9231.

Kyolic (see Garlic)
Wakunaga of America Ltd., 23501 Madero, Mission Viejo, CA 92691. Phone: (714) 855-2776.

Ayurvedic herbs
Ayur-Veda Herb Co., Nature Herbs (a division of Twinlabs), Box 336, Orem, UT 84059.

American Association of Ayurvedic Medicine, Box 282, Farifield, IA 52556. Phone: (515) 472-5866. For orders: 800 255-8322.

Benzaldehyde
Essential Oil Source - Phone: 800 289-8427.

Dr. Hans Nieper. Sedan Strasse 21, 3000 Hannover 1, Germany. Phone: 49-511-348-08-08.

Butyric Acid
Allergy Research Group, PO Box 489/400 Preda Street, San Lenadro, CA 94577-0489. Phone: 800 545-9960.

Ecological Formulas, 1061-B Shary Circle, Concord, CA 94518. Phone: 800 888-4585. (510) 827-2636 Fax (510) 676-9231.

ProBiologic Inc. West Willows Technology Ctr., 14714 NE 87th Street, Redmond, WA 98052. Phone: 800 678-8218.

Antineoplastons (BURZYNSKI):
BURNZYNSKI RESEARCH INSTITUTE, Outpatients Clinic: 6221 Corporate Drive, Houston, TX 77036. (713) 777-8233.

Vitamin C
LINUS PAULING INSTITUTE OF SCIENCE AND MEDICINE 440 Page Mill Road, Palo Alto, CA 94306. (415) 327-4064.

Allergy Research Group, P.O. Box 489/400 Preda Street, San Lenadro, CA 94577-0489. Phone: (415) 639-4572 or 800 545-9960.

Ecological Formulas, 1061-B Shary Circle, Concord, CA 94518. Phone: 800 888-4585. (510) 827-2636 Fax (510) 676-9231.

Miller Pharmacal Group 4563 Prime Parkway Dr. P.O. Box 1297 Mc Henry, Illinois, 60050-1297. Phone: 800 323-2935.

GY&N Nutrient Pharmacology P.O. Box 2252, Carlsbad, CA 92018 (619) 434-6360, 800 445-2122, Fax (619) 434-0816.

Canthaxanthin
Wholesale Nutrition, P.O. Box 3345, Saratoga, CA 95070-1345 Phone: 800 325-2664.

Chaparral
Tri-Sun North Americal, 109 1\2 Broadway, Box 1606, Fargo, ND 58107. Phone: (701) 234-9654. Jason Winter's Tea contains red clover and Chinese herbs in addition to chaparral. Chaparral tea as a douche; for the precancerous condition, cervical dysplasia - four capsules in a quart of water, covered for fifteen minutes. Strain out the particles and allow it to cool.

Chelation
Chelation should only be administered by a trained professional. See the list under Professional Resource categories for members of The American College of Advances in Medicine.

Miller Pharmacal Group 4563 Prime Parkway Dr. P.O. Box 1297 Mc Henry, Illinois, 60050-1297. Phone: 800 323-2935. Fax (815) 344-2378.

GY&N Nutrient Pharmacology P.O. Box 2252, Carlsbad, CA 92018 (619) 434-6360, 800 445-2122, Fax (619) 434-0816.

Chinese Medicines
Chinatowns of larger cities.

Nuherbs Co., 3820 Penniman Ave., Oakland, CA 94619. Phone: 800-233-4307. In California: (415) 534-HERB. Fax: (415) 534-3484.

Tashi Enterprises, 3252 Ramona St., Pinole CA 94564. Phone: 800 888-9998.

Mrs. Tsong's Herbal Tonic Soups 379A Clementina St., San Francisco, CA 94103. Phone: (415) 441-5505.

Chlorophyll
Life Extension Foundation. Phone: 800 544-0577

Tri-Sun North America, 109 1/2 Broadway, Box 1606, Fargo, ND 58107. Phone: 800 447-0235 or (701) 234-9654.

DHEA (Dehydroepiandrosterone)

College Pharmacy 833 N. Tejon St. Colorado Springs, CO 80903. Phone: 800 748-2263.

Belmar Pharmacy 8015 W. Alameda Ave. Lakewood, CO 80226. Phone: 800 525-9473.

DMSO

Natural Health Center, PO Box N-8941, Third Terrace, Collins Avenue, Nassau, Bahamas. Phone: (809) 326-6565.

Michael B. Schachter, MD, PC, and Associates, Two Executive Boulevard, Suite 202, Suffern, NY 10901. Phone: (914) 368-4700.

Rimso-50 Research Industries Corporation Pharmaceutical Division, 6864 South 300 West, Midvale, UT 84047.

Electromagnetic Devices

Magne-tec Enterprises Inc., 14 Connie Crescent, Unit 2, Concord, Ontario, L4K 2W8. Phone: (416) 669-1154.

Alpha Energy Products, Inc., 7027 SW 87th Court, Miami, FL 33173. Phone (305) 271-8815.

Enzymes

Ecological Formulas, 1061-B Shary Circle, Concord, CA 94518. Phone: 800 888-4585, (510) 827-2636 Fax (510) 676-9231.

Advanced Medical Nutrition, Inc P.O. Box 5012, 2247 National Ave. Hayward, CA 94540.

Ernst T. Krebs, Jr., DSc, John Beard Memorial Foundation, P.O. Box 685, San Francisco, CA 94101. Phone: (415) 824-1067.

Nicholas Gonzalez MD, 730 Park Avenue, New York, NY 10021. Phone: (212) 535-3993.

Mr. David Sauder, Nutri Supplies, 1020 Stony Battery Road,

Lancaster, PA 17601. Phone: 800 999-2700.

NutriCology, Inc., Allergy Research Group, P.O. Box 489, San Leandro, CA 94577-0489. Phone: 800 782-4274.

C.P.W. Rahlstedt, Box 73 0527, D-W-2000 Hamburg, Germany.

Source for Wobenzym and Wobe-mugos. Wakunaga of America Ltd., 2305 Madero, Mission Viejo, CA 92691. Phone: (714) 855-2776.

Scientific Consulting Service, Inc., 5725 Chelton Drive, Oakland, California, 94611. Phone: (415) 531-3246.

Emerson Ecologics, 14 Newtown Road, Acton, MA 01720. Phone: 1 800 654 4432 or 1 (508) 263-7238.

Staff of Life P.O. Box 1268 Duvall, WA 98019. Phone: 800 743-7531 Fax (206) 788-1564.

Miller Pharmacal Group 4563 Prime Parkway Dr. P.O. Box 1297 Mc Henry, Illinois, 60050-1297. Phone: 800 323-2935 Fax (815) 344-2378.

GY&N Nutrient Pharmacology P.O. Box 2252, Carlsbad, CA 92018. Phone: (619) 434-6360, 800 445-2122.

Essiac Formula
Claude Corson c/o Totem Products, P.O. Box 638, White Pigeon, MI 49099. Phone: (616) 483-7644. Burdock root is available as a botanical liquid extract or fresh freeze-dried from The Eclectic Institute.

Essential Fatty Acids
Miller Pharmacal Group 4563 Prime Parkway Dr. P.O. Box 1297 Mc Henry, Illinois, 60050-1297. Phone: 800 323-2935.

Fiber
Advanced Medical Nutrition, Inc P.O. Box 5012, 2247 National

Ave. Hayward, CA 94540.

Fish Oil (Fatty Acids)
Ecological Formulas, 1061-B Shary Circle, Concord, CA 94518.
Phone: 800 888-4585. (510) 827-2636 Fax (510) 676-9231.

Advanced Medical Nutrition, Inc P.O. Box 5012, 2247 National
Ave. Hayward, CA 94540.

Miller Pharmacal Group 4563 Prime Parkway Dr., P.O. Box
1297 Mc Henry, Illinois, 60050-1297. Phone: 800 323-2935 Fax
(815) 344-2378.

Aquaculture Marketing Service, 356 W. Redview Dr., Monroe,
UT 84754. Phone: (801) 527-4528.

GY&N Nutrient Pharmacology P.O. Box 2252, Carlsbad, CA
92018 (619) 434-6360, 800 445-2122, Fax (619) 434-0816.

Mountain Ark Trading Company, Fayetteville, AR 72701.
Phone: 800 643-8909.

Flutamide
Patient Advocates for Advanced Cancer Treatments, Inc. 1143
Parmalee NW, Grand Rapids, MI 49504. Phone: (616)
453-1477.

Garlic
Advanced Medical Nutrition, Inc P.O. Box 5012, 2247 National
Ave. Hayward, CA 94540.

Miller Pharmacal Group 4563 Prime Parkway Dr., P.O. Box
1297 Mc Henry, Illinois 60050-1297. Phone: 800 323-2935, Fax
(815) 344-2378.

Arizona Natural Products, Michael Hanna, 8281 E. Evans Road,
104 Scottsdale, AZ 85260.

Pleasant Groves Farms. Ed or Wynette Sills, P.O. Box 636,
Pleasant Grove, CA 95668. Phone: (916) 655-3391.

Walnut Acres, Walnut Acres Road, Penns Creek, PA 17862. Phone: 800 433-3998.

Germanium
Advanced Medical Nutrition, Inc P.O. Box 5012, 2247 National Ave. Hayward, CA 94540.

Allergy Research Group, P.O. Box 489/400 Preda Street, San Lenadro, CA 94577-0489. Phone: 800 545-9960.

Miller Pharmacal Group 4563 Prime Parkway Dr., P.O. Box 1297 Mc Henry, Illinois, 60050-1297. Phone: 800 323-2935.

Ginseng
Jin Han International Inc., Brooklyn NY 11211.

Pacific Foods Inc., Los Angeles, CA 90011.

New York's Chinatown (Just about anywhere)!

Green Tea
Wah Yin Hong Enterprises, 232 Canal Street, New York, NY 10013. Phone: (212) 941-8954.

The American Health Foundation, 1 Dana Road, Valhalla, NY 10595. Phone: (914) 592-2600, Fax: (914) 592-6317.

Glandulars and Herbals
Allergy Research Group, P.O. Box 489/400 Preda Street, San Lenadro, CA 94577-0489. Phone: 800 545-9960.

Ecological Formulas, 1061-B Shary Circle, Concord, CA 94518. Phone: 800 888-4585.

GY&N Nutrient Pharmacology P.O. Box 2252, Carlsbad, CA 92018 (619) 434-6360, (800) 445-2122, Fax (619) 434-0816

Bio Life 1717 N. Bayshore Drive #1836 Miami, FL 33132 (305) 375-0200 Fax (305) 375-0009.

Miller Pharmacal Group 4563 Prime Parkway Dr., P.O. Box 1297 Mc Henry, Illinois, 60050-1297 (800) 323-2935 Fax (815) 344-2378.

Herbs
Phyto-Pharmica, P.O. Box 1348, Green Bay, Wisconsin 54305, Phone: 1 800 553-2370 Fax: (414) 437-4087.

Eclectic Institute, 11231 SE Market Street, Portland OR 97216. Phone: (503) 256-4330 or 1 800 332-4372.

Yerba Prima, P.O. Box 2569, Oakland, CA 94614.

Futurebiotics, 48 Elliot Street, Brattleboro, VT 05301. Phone: Karen Reardon at 1 800 367-5433.

Solaray, 2815 Industrial Drive, Ogden, Utah 84401-9983.

Ecological Formulas, 1061-B Shary Circle, Concord, CA 94518. Phone: 800 888-4585.

GY&N Nutrient Pharmacology P.O. Box 2252, Carlsbad, CA 92018 (619) 434-6360, 800 445-2122, Fax (619) 434-0816.

Herbs and Spices
Eclectic Institute 11231 S.E. Market Street, Portland, OR 97216. Phone: 800-332-4372. An affiliate of the National College of Naturopathic Medicine. They also make herbal tinctures. Catalogue available. Provides freeze-dried extracts.

Homeopathics
Standard Homeopathic Co., 210 W. 131st St., Box 61067, Los Angeles, CA 90061. Phone: 800 624-9659 or (213) 321-4284. Fax: (213) 516-8579.

HOM. INT. P.O. Box 410240, D-7500 Karlsruhe, Germany. Phone: (49) 721 4093 228 Fax: (49) 721 4093-602-334.
Similia Laboratories, Inc. Editorial Staff: Luc Chaltin, ND.

Hoxsey Formula
Bio-Medical Center clinic is in Tijuana, P.O. Box 727, General
Ferreira 615, Col Juarez, Tijuana, B.C. Mexico. Phone:
706-648-9011.

Lenex Laboratory, PO Box 358, Watersmeet, MI 49969, Phone:
(906) 358-4802. Product similar to Hoxsey's external salve.

Hydrazine sulfate
Dr. Joseph Gold, Syracuse Research Institute, 600 East Genesee
Street, Syracuse, NY 13202. Phone: (315) 472-6616.

Ms. Donna Schuster, Great Lakes Metabolics, 1724 Hiawatha
Court, NE, Rochester, MN 55904. Phone: (507) 288-2348.

Syracuse Cancer Research Institute Inc., Presidentail Plaza, 600
East Genesee Street, Syracuse, NY 13202. (315) 472-6616.

Iscador
Society for Cancer Research (Swiss Anthroposophic Organisa-
tion). in Arlesheim, Switzerland.

Rudolf Steiner Fellowship Foundation, 41 Hungry Hollow
Road, Spring Valley, NY 10977. Phone: (914) 356-8494/
914-6835.

The Lukas Klinik CH-4144 Arlesheim, Switzerland. Phone:
41-61-72-3333.

Dr. H. B. von Laue, Klinik Oschelbronn, Am Eichhof, 753
Niefern-Oschelbronn 2, Germany. Phone: 0 72 33 6 80. Fax: 0
72 33 6 81 10.

Lactobacillus
Allergy Research Group, P.O. Box 489/400 Preda Street, San
Lenadro, CA 94577-0489. Phone: 800 545-9960.

Advanced Medical Nutrition, Inc P.O. Box 5012, 2247 National
Ave. Hayward, CA 94540.

Ecological Formulas, 1061-B Shary Circle, Concord, CA 94518. Phone: 800 888-4585.

Staff of Life P.O. Box 1268 Duvall, WA 98019. Phone: 800 743-7531 Fax (206) 788-1564.

A.R. Donohoe 1267 Southeast Ave. Tallmadge, Ohio (216) 434-2927.

Miller Pharmacal Group 4563 Prime Parkway Dr., P.O. Box 1297. Mc Henry, Illinois, 60050-1297. Phone: 800 323-2935.

GY&N Nutrient Pharmacology P.O. Box 2252, Carlsbad, CA 92018. Phone: (619) 434-6360, 800 445-2122.

Urea
David Steenblock, DO, 22821 Lake Forest Drive, Suite 114, El Toro, CA 92630. Phone: (714) 770-9616.

Vincent Speckhart, MD, 902 Graydon Avenue, Suite 2, Norfolk, VA 23507. Phone: (804) 622-0014. or (804) 622-5333.

Bio-Tech of Fayetteville, P.O. Box 1992, Fayetteville, AR 72702. Phone: 800 345-1199 or (501) 443-9148. Will ship direct to patients, if doctor so directs.

Pharmaceuticals International, 539 Telegraph Canyon Road 227, Chula Vista, CA 92010. Phone: 800 365-3698.

Dr. Evangelos D. Danopoulos, 12 Rigillis Str., 106-74 Athens, Greece. Phone: 011-301-721-5318.

Guillermo J. Panafox, M.D. 3003 Gobernor Lane, Tijuana, Mexico Contact: Sierra Clinics P.O. Box 3187 Walnut Creek, CA 94598.

Shark Cartilage
Ecological Formulas, 1061-B Shary Circle, Concord, CA 94518. Phone: 800 888-4585.

Allergy Research Group, P.O. Box 489/400 Preda Street, San Lenadro, CA 94577-0489. Phone: (415) 639-4572.

Squalene
GY&N Nutrient Pharmacology P.O. Box 2252, Carlsbad, CA 92018. Phone: (619) 434-6360, 800 445-2122.

Linseed Oil
Allergy Research Group, P.O. Box 489/400 Preda Street, San Lenadro, CA 94577-0489. Phone: 800 545-9960.

GY&N Nutrient Pharmacology P.O. Box 2252, Carlsbad, CA 92018. Phone: (619) 434-6360, 800 445-2122.

New Dimensions Distributors, Inc., (C-Leinosan) 16548 E. Laser St., Bldg. A-7, Fountain Hills, AZ 85268, 1 800 624-7114.

Megace
Dr. Jamie H. von Roenn, Department of Hematology/Oncology, Northwestern University Medical School, 233 East Erie, Room 700, Chicago, IL 60611. Phone: (312) 908-5284.

Dr. Patricia A. Johnson, MD, Carle Clinic, University of Illinois, 602 West University, Urbana, IL 61801. Phone: (217) 383-3010.

Methylene blue
Star Pharmacuticals, 1990 N.W. 44th Street, Pompano Beach, FL 33064.

Webcon Pharmaceuticals, P.O. Box 6380, Fort Worth, TX 76115. Manufactures Urised (reg), contains methylene blue Phone: (817) 293-0450.

Health Enhancement Services, Inc. 30 West Mashta Drive, Key Biscayne, FL 33149. Phone: (305) 365-9000.

Mu-er
Wah Yin Hong Enterprises, Canal Street, New York, NY

10013. Phone: (212) 941-8954.

Mushrooms
Maitake Products, Inc. P.O. Box 1354, Paramus, NJ 07653. Phone: 800 747-7418 or (201) 612-0097.

Onconase
New York Medical College, Department of Oncology, Munger Pavilion, Room 250, Valhalla, NY 10595. Patent Contact: Dr. Mittleman or Dr. Chun. Phone: (914) 993-8374.

The Thompson Cancer Survival Center, Knoxville, TN. Principle Investigator: Dr. John Costanzi Patent contact: Jan Miller, Phone: (615) 541-4966.

Alfacell Corporation, 25 Belleville Avenue, Bloomfield, NJ 07003. Phone: (201) 748-0882. Fax: (201) 748-1355.

Ozone Equipment
O$_3$ Tech Mfg., Jim Brown, 1101 So. Rogers Circle Boca Raton, FL 33431.

Dr, Hansler OZONOSAN, Nordring 8, 76473 Iffezhelm, Germany. Tele: 07229/30 46 0 Fax: 07229/30 46 30.

Pau d'Arco
Ecological Formulas, 1061-B Shary Circle, Concord, CA 94518. Phone: 800 888-4585.

Lindberg Nutrition, Torrance, CA Phone: 800 338-797.

Ubiquinone (Co-enzyme Q-10)
Ecological Formulas, 1061-B Shary Circle, Concord, CA 94518. Phone: 800 888-4585.

Allergy Research Group, P.O. Box 489/400 Preda Street, San Lenadro, CA 94577-0489. Phone: (415) 639-4572.

Miller Pharmacal Group 4563 Prime Parkway Dr., P.O. Box 1297 Mc Henry, Illinois, 60050. Phone: 800 323-2935.

Advanced Medical Nutrition, Inc P.O. Box 5012, 2247 National Ave. Hayward, CA 94540.

Futurebiotics, 48 Elliot Str., Brattleboro, VT 05301. Phone: 800 367-5433.

GY&N Nutrient Pharmacology P.O. Box 2252, Carlsbad, CA 92018. Phone: (619) 434-6360, 800 445-2122, Fax (619) 434-0816.

Spices
Tumeric and other spices are available in most markets and health food stores.

Vitamin - Minerals
Advanced Medical Nutrition, Inc P.O. Box 5012, 2247 National Ave. Hayward, CA 94540.

Ecological Formulas, 1061-B Shary Circle, Concord, CA 94518. Phone: 800 888-4585.

Allergy Research Group, P.O. Box 489/400 Preda Street, San Lenadro, CA 94577-0489. Phone: 800 545-9960.

Miller Pharmacal Group 4563 Prime Parkway Dr., P.O. Box 1297 Mc Henry, Illinois, 60050-1297. Phone: 800 323-2935.

GY&N Nutrient Pharmacology P.O. Box 2252, Carlsbad, CA 92018. Phone: (619) 434-6360, 800 445-2122..

PHARMACEUTICALS -

That are sometimes difficult to obtain in smaller cities and towns. Professionals only. Some fill prescriptions.

Belmar Pharmacy, 8015 W. Alameda Ave., Suite 100, Lakewood, CO 80226. Phone: 800 525-9473.

College Pharmacy, 833 N. Tejon St., Colorado Springs, CO 80903. Phone: 800 748-2263.

The Mail Order Pharmacy 3170 Federal Highway - Suite 104B Lighthouse Point, FL 33064. Phone: 800 822-5388, (305) 786-1304.

INFORMATION SOURCES

International Societies
Intl. Society for Preventive Oncology, 217, East 85th St. 303 New York, NY 10028. Phone: (212) 534-4991.

World Institute of Ecology and Cancer, Rue de Fripiers 24 bis B-1000, Bruxelles, Belgium. Phone: 32 2 219 08 30.

European Society for Psychosocial Oncology, Service d'Hematologie, Hotel-Dieu, Place du Parvis, Notre-Dame, F-75181 Paris CEDEX 04 France.

International Psycho-oncology Project, Bergstrasse 10, D-2900, Oldenburg, Germany. Phone: (49 441)1 31 47.

World Health Org., Melanoma Program Instit. Nazionale Tumori, Via Veneziana 1, I-20133 Milano, Italy. Phone: 39 2 29 39 92.

Intl. Comm. for Protection Against Environmental Mutagens & Carcinogens, Medical Biological Laboratory, TNO, P.O. Box 45, 2280 AA Rijswijk, Netherlands.

INFORMATION, RESOURCES, REFERRALS AND ACTION GROUPS YOU CAN JOIN

Life Extension Foundation 2490 Griffin Rd., Fort Lauderdale FL 33312. Phone 1 - 800 841-5433 (305) 966-4886.

American Assoc. of Orthomolecular Medicine, 7375 Kingsway Burnaby, British Columbia, V3N3B5 Canada.

American College of Advances in Medicine, 231 Verdugo Drive, Suite 204, Laguna Hills, CA 92653. Phone: (714) 583-7666.

Alternative Cancer Therapies 2043 N. Berendo Street Los Angeles, CA 90027 (203) 663-7801.

Arlin J. Brown Information Center, P.O. Box 251, Ft. Belvoir, VA 22060. Phone: (703) 451-8638.

Cancer Control Society, 2043 N. Berendo St., Los Angeles, CA 90027. Phone: (213) 664-7801.

Can Help, 3111 Paradis Bay Road Port Ludlow, WA 98365 Phone: (206) 437-2291.

Comm. for Freedom of Choice in Medicine, 1180 Walnut Ave., Chula Vista, CA 92011. Phone: 800-227-4473/ Fax: (619) 429-8004.

European Institute for Orthomolecular Sciences, P.O. Box 420, 3740 A.K. Baarn, Holland.

Foundation for Advancement in Cancer Therapy, Box 1242, Old Chelsea Sta. New York, NY 10113. Phone:(212) 741-2790.

Gerson Institute, PO Box 430, Bonita, CA 91908. Phone: (619) 267-1150/ Fax: (619) 267-6441.

Intl. Academy of Nutrition and Preventive Medicine, P.O. Box 18433, Asheville, NC 28814. Phone: (704) 258-3243/ Fax: (704) 251-9206.

Intl. Assn. of Cancer Victors & Friends, 7740 W. Manchester Ave., No. 110, Playa del Rey, CA 90293. Phone: (213) 822-5032. Fax: (213) 822-5132.

We Can Do! 1800 Augusta, Ste. 150, Houston, TX 77057. Phone: (713) 780-1057.

Ontario Naturopathic Association 4195 Dundas Street West - Suite 213 West Toronto, Ontario M9X 1X8 Canada. Phone: (416) 234-5560.

People Against Cancer, Box 10, Otho, IA 50569. Phone: 1 (515) 972-4444. Fax: (515) 972-4415.

Simonton Cancer Center, P.O. Box 890, Pacific Palisades, CA 90272. Phone: (213) 459-4434.

Biological Homepathic Industries, 11600 Cochiti S.E., Albuquerque, New Mexico 87123. Phone: 800 621-7644 or (505) 293-3843 Fax: (505) 275-1672.

Wright/Gaby Nutrition Institute, P.O. Box 21535, Baltimore, Md. 21208.

Academy of Orthomolescular Medicine/Huxley Institute, P.O. Box 1731, Boca Raton, FL 33429.

American Academy of Environmental Medicine, P.O. Box 16106, Denver, CO 80216.

Journal of Orthomolescular Medicine/CFS, 16 Florence Ave., Toronto, Ontario, M2N 1E9, Canada.. Phone: (416) 773-2117.

Price-Pottenger Nutrition Foundation, P.O. Box 2614, La Mesa, CA 92044-2614.

National Health Federation, Legislative Advocates, Box 528, Gainesville, VA 22065-0528.

Coalition for Alternatives in Nutrition and Healthcare, Inc. (CANAH), PO Box B-12, Richlandtown, PA 18955.

Belmar Pharmacy, 8015 W. Alameda Ave., Suite 100, Lakewood, CO 80226. Phone: 800 525-9473.

College Pharmacy, 833 N. Tejon St., Colorado Springs, CO 80903. Phone: 800 748-2263.

Villain Limited, P.O. Box 467, Glasgow, G52 2UF, Scotland. Phone: 041 425 1930.

Society of Complementary Medicine in London, 31 Weymouth Street, London, W1N 3FJ. Phone: 071 436 0821.

Homeopathic Education and Research, 5916 Chabot Crest, Oakland, CA 94618. Phone: (415) 420-8791.

Life Extension Foundation 2490 Griffin Rd., Fort Lauderdale FL 33312. Phone 1 - 800 841-5433 (305) 966-4886.

James W. Prescott, Ph.D. Biobehavioural Systems, 5175 Luigi Terrace 35, San Diego, CA 92122.

ALLOPATHIC
(ESTABLISHMENT MEDICINE) TREATMENT

NATIONAL CANCER INSTITUTE, (800) 4-CANCER.

INFORMATION AND REFERRALS FOR
ALTERNATIVE TREATMENT CENTERS

In Tijuana, Mexico, contact; ANDREW McNAUGHTON, Tel. 011-52-66-300-481 or HUGUES BELLEVIEW, M.D. Tel. 619-469-1360 (Cal.) 011-52-66-301-966 (Mex.)

AMERICAN BIOLOGICS - MEXICO S.A. MEDICAL CENTER, 1180 Walnut Avenue, Chula Vista, CA 92011. Phone: (619) 429-8200, 800 227-4458 or 800 227-4473 (CA) **(Be sure the Laetrile is mixed in front of you).**

NEVADA CLINIC 2300 W. Sahara, Las Vegas, NV 89103. Phone: (702) 871-2700 or 800 641-6661.

AMERICAN INTERNATIONAL HOSPITAL Shiloh and Emmans Avenue, Zion, IL 60099. (708) 872-4561 800 For Help.

SAM BAXAS, MD., Baxamed Switzerland Medical Center, Realpstrasse 83, CH-4054 Basel, Switzerland. (061) 302-9066: Telex: 965 137 Buph ch. Fax: (061) 301 3872.

ONTARIO NATUROPATHIC ASSOCIATION 4195 Dundas Street West - Suite 213, West Toronto, Ontario, M9X 1X8, Canada. (416) 234-5560.

FINN ANDERSON, MD., Hum Legaarden Clinic, NY Strandveg 11, DK 3050 Humleback, Denmark.

HANS A. NIEPER, MD., Inpatient Clinic, Paracelsus Klinik at Siberscem Oertzeweg 24, 3012 Langenhagen, Germany. 011-49-511-348-08-08 Outpatient Office: Sedan Strasse 21, 3000 Hanover 1, Germany. 011-49-511-348-08-08.

SIICHI KAWACHI, MD., 7-3-8 Ginza Chuo-ku, Tokyo, Japan. 03-572-5455.

BIRCHER-BRENNER PRIVATKLINIK, Keltenstrasse 48, CH 8044 Zurich, Switzerland. 011-41-1251-68-90.

R. ARNOLD SMITH, MD, 701 Alcorn Drive, Corinth, MS 38834. Phone: (601) 286-4252.

NICHOLAS J. GONZALEZ, MD, 737 Park Avenue, New York, NY 10021. Phone: (212) 535-3993.

BIOLOGICAL THERAPY INSTITUTE Hospital Drive, Franklin, TN 37064. Phone: (615) 790-7535.

RUTH CILENTO, MD, 1 Trackson Street, Alderly, Brisbane 4051, Australia. 07-352-6634

BRISTOL CANCER HELP CENTRE, Grove House, Cornwallis Grove, Clifton, Bristol, B28 4PG, England. 011-44-272-743216.

IMMUNO-AUGMENTATIVE THERAPY CENTRE, P.O. Box F-2689, Freeport, Grand Bahama Island, Bahamas. (809) 352-7455/6.

COLEY'S TOXINS:
CANCER RESEARCH INSTITUTE, 133 East 58 Street, New

York, NY 10022, 800 223-7874 or 800 522-5022 (in New York).

THE GERSON METHOD:
GERSON INSTITUTE, P.O. Box 430, Bonita, CA 92002. (619) 267-1150.

HYDRAZINE SULFATE THERAPY:
JOSEPH GOLD, MD, Presidential Plaza, 600 East Genesee Street, Syracuse, NY 13202. (315) 472-6616.

LAETRILE AND METABOLIC THERAPY See recommendation at the beginning of this section.

IMMUNO-AUGMENTATIVE THERAPY AND OTHER TREATMENTS AND PATIENT'S RIGHTS:
PEOPLE AGAINST CANCER Box 10, Otho, IA 50569-0010 Phone: (515) 972-4444.

LEGAL/POLITICAL STRUGGLES IN THE CANCER FIELD:
PATIENT RIGHTS LEGAL ACTION FUND, 202 West 78 Street #3E, New York, NY 10024.

DENTAL AMALGAM TOXICITY REMOVAL:
HAL A. HUGGINS, DDS,MS, P.O. Box 2589, Colorado Springs, CO 80901. (719) 548-1600.

DAVID C. KENNEDY, DDS, 2425 3 Avenue, San Diego, CA 92101. (619) 231-1624.

W. WAYNE KING, DDM, 1200 Rosewall Road, SE, VPI Corp Building 2 level, Marjetta, GA 30062. (404) 426-0288.

****

ABOUT THE AUTHOR...

CURRICULUM VITAE

ROBERT E. WILLNER, M.D., Ph.D.

EDUCATIONAL BACKGROUND

1987	University for Humanistic Studies (accredited) Las Vegas, Nevada **Degree: Doctor of Humane Letters (Ph.D, in Nutrition)**
1951-1955	New York Medical College New York City, New York **Degree: Doctor of Medicine**
1948-1951	New York University College of Arts and Sciences, University Heights, New York City, New York **Degree: Bachelor of Arts** (Major: Psychology Minor: Biochemistry, Music)
1947-1948	University of Southern California Los Angeles, California Freshman Year toward B.A. degree
1943-1947	Music and Art High School New York City, New York **Degree: High School Diploma,** Music Major

POSTGRADUATE ACTIVITIES

1987	**American Board of Pain Management Specialties Fellow (FABPMS-C)**
	American Academy of Neurologic and Orthopedic Medicine and
Surgery,	
	Fellow (FAANaOS-Cm)
	American Board of Legal Analysis in Medicine and Surgery, Fellow (FABLAAMS)
1983	Chelation Therapy Workshop The American Academy of Medical Preventics Reno, Nevada
1979	**The American Board of Family Physicians Recertification**
1976	Postgraduate Institute for Emergency Medical Care University of California, San Diego
	"Our Inner Conflicts" CE208 School of Continuing Studies University of Miami, Miami, Florida
1974	Second World Symposium On Acupuncture And Chinese Medicine The American Society of Chinese Medicine
1973	The American Association of Sex Educators and Counselors, The American University **Certificate in Sex Education**
1972	**American Board of Family Medicine Diplomate (ABFM-D)**
1961	**Arroyo Academy of Advanced Hypnosis Certification**
1959	**Florida Board of Medical Examiners Certification**
1956	**School of Aviation Medicine Basic Certification**

1955   National Board of Medical Examiners

POSTGRADUATE PROFESSIONAL CAREER

1959-1989   Private Practice of Medicine, North Miami Beach, Florida
1955-1959   United States Air Force, General Medical Officer, Chief of Emergency
            Service, Chief of Obstetrical Service, Base Psychiatric Officer
1955-1956   Memorial Hospital, Phoenix, Arizona **Internship**
1954-1955   Flower and Fifth Avenue Hospital, New York City, New York **Internship**
            Bird S. Coler Hospital for Physical Medicine and Rehabilitation
            Internship

SOCIETY MEMBERSHIPS

1989-1991   American Physicians Associations
1985-1991   American College of Advancement in Medicine
1984-1991   American Academy of Neurological and Orthopedic Medicine and
            Surgery 1962-1987 Southern Medical Association
1983   International Association for the Study of Pain
1983   International Laser Research Academy
1979   German Academy of Auricular Medicine
1979   American Society of Bariatric Physicians
1975   South Florida Council of Medical Staffs
1972   American Institute of Hypnosis
1960   American Medical Association
            Florida Medical Association Dade County Medical Association
            American Academy of Family Physicians
            Florida Academy of Family Physicians
            Dade County Academy of Family Physicians 1952
            Phi Delta Epsilon Medical Fraternity

HOSPITAL ASSOCIATIONS

1960-1989   Parkway Regional Medical Center, North Miami Beach, Florida - Senior
            Attending Physician

HONORS AND SPECIAL ACTIVITIES

1990-1991   American College of Advancement in Medicine   Sargent At
              (Board Of Directors)   Arms

1989-1991   American Physicians Association   Executive
                                                               Secretary

1988-1991   American Academy of Advancementin Medicine   Board of
                                                               Directors

1987-1991   American Board of Pain Management Specialties   Professor &
                                                               Chairman

1983-1984   International Laser Research Academy   President
            Linda Georgian Television Medical Show   Advisor

1982-1984   Conference on Holistic Medicine Walter Reed   Lecturer

Hospital, Wash. D.C.

1977-1984	Concept House Drug Rehabilitation Miami, Florida	Medical Director
1981-1982	Medical Research Laboratories Chicago, Illinois	Medical Director
1980-1982	Oleda Inc. New York City, New York	Medical Director
1980	The Funhouse Motion Company "The Funhouse"	Medical Consultant
	McGill University Medical School Preceptor	
1978-1980	Florida International University Univ. of Miami School of Medicine	Lecturer Lecturer
1979	Paramount Pictures Corporation "Spanner's Key"	Medical Consultant
1962-1979	Dade County Medical Association	Lecturer
1978	Truman Van Dyke Company Medical "Woman In White"	Consultant
1978	Nurse Practitioner Program University of Miami	Preceptor
1977-1978	National Acupuncture Research Society	**Board of Directors**
1974-1977	National Acupuncture Research Society	Faculty
1977	Motion Picture "The Champ"	Medical Consultant
1972-1976	Spectrum House Rehabilitation Center, Miami, Florida	Medical Director
1975	South Florida Council of Medical Staffs	**Secretary**
1974	Florida Academy of Family Physicians	**Vice-Pres.**
	American Medical Association Physician Recognition Award American Academy of Family Physicians, Award Certificate	
1968-1974	Dade County Academy of Family Physicians	**Board of Directors**
1968-1974	Florida Academy of Family Physicians	**Board of Directors**
1973	American Academy of Family Physicians	Charter Fellow
1972	Parkway General Hospital Certificate of Appreciation	Chief of Staff

1971	Parkway General Hospital Dept. of Family Practice	Chairman
1970-1971	Dade County Academy of Family Practice	**President**
1966	City of North Miami Beach, Certificate of Recognition and Appreciation	
1955	Cor et Manus New York Medical College	Award of Distinction
1951	National Student Association New York University	Senior Delegate
	Perstare et Praestare New York University	Honor Society
	Student Council New York University	

POSTGRADUATE EDUCATION

1976-1987	Parkway Regional Medical Center ContinuingEducation Seminars - Forty credits per annum
1986	American Academy of Neurologic and Orthopedic Medicine and Surgery "Communication SkillsWorkshops" Fifty hours, Las Vegas, Nevada
1986	"Allergy In Practice" Roche Biomedical Laboratories Miami, Florida
1975	Advanced Acupuncture Workshop, National Acupuncture Research Society
1974	Intermediate Acupuncture Workshop, National Acupuncture Research Society
1972	Family Practice Review Course, University of Alabama, Schooll of Medicine

PUBLICATIONS

1994	**"The Ultimate Deception"** Peltec Publishing Co. Inc.
	"The Cancer Solution" Peltec Publishing Co. Inc.
1984	**"The Pleasure Principle Diet"** Prentice-Hall, May 1985 ISBN O-13-683442-6 (225 pages)
	"The Effect of Low Power on Osteoarthritis of The Hands" IV World Pain Congress Seattle, Washington 1978
	"Communicating With The Depressed Elderly Patients" Co-author: Marcia Willner Continuing Education, November 1978
1974	**"Acupuncture Desk Reference"**
	"Touching Is ..."
	"Acupuncture Wall Charts"
	"Professional Acupuncture Seminar Workbook"

LECTURES

Over two hundred and fifty presentations have been given to the profession and the public. Many radio and television appearances have been taped. A list of most of the lectures is available on request. Some audio and video tapes are also available.

PERSONAL DATA

Date of Birth: June 21, 1929
Place of Birth: New York City, New York

RECENT ACTIVITIES

1989 - 1993   Retired from the practice of medicine to pursue research in Cancer, "AIDS", Chronic Degenerative Diseases and solutions to ecological problems.

1993   Cydel Medical Center for Advanced Therapies,
                Consulting Executive Medical Director to update and expand therapeutic program.

                Life-Line Consultants
                Executive Director Independent Guidance to the Availability of Therapeutic Solutions to Cancer, "AIDS" and Chronic Degenerative Diseases"

THE CANCER SOLUTION

AN INVITATION TO SHARE
YOUR KNOWLEDGE

I have tried to present an easy to understand and complete beacon in THE CANCER SOLUTION. However, there are many answers to achieving and maintaining optimum health that are not easy to find or not accessible.

If you are aware of therapies, techniques, resources and practitioners that I have not included, write to me in care of the publisher, and it will be included in the next addition.

... and to prove I mean it ...

After I sent the manuscript to the publisher, a friend sent me an article from THE TOWNSEND LETTER FOR DOCTORS, an excellent publication. The article was entitled, "Two More Unused, Anti-cancer Treatments" by Wayne Thompson. The publisher agreed to add it at the end.

TREATMENT 1 - HYDROCHLORIC ACID

Thompson writes of the Hydrochloric Acid Therapy (HCL) developed by Burr Ferguson, M.D., in the 1920's. Following an article in Medical World, reports from all over the world told of incredible recoveries from infections and cancer using HCL. Dr. Ferguson used a dilution of one part HCL to 500 - 1500 cc of sterile water, injecting 10cc intravenously and repeating it daily as the condition indicated. HCL is used today in Mexico and elsewhere. **Many physicians who administer chelation therapy include HCL in the I.V. drip (see the chapter on Chelation).**

In 1935, a Dr. Guy added benzoic acid to the therapy. He published reports on success in the treatment of epithelioma, myoma (fibroids) of the uterus and Hodgkin's disease. Dr. Guy's formulation consisted of:

Oral solution: Acidibenzoic Acid, 10 gm; Alcohol 95%, 90 cc; Saturated solution of silicic acid in dilute HCL, USP clor rubrum, Q.S. added to 120cc. Dose; 15 drops in 8 oz. of distilled water, 3 to 5 times a day. This solution can be used as a throat spray or for topical application. For intravenous administration: OMIT the silicic acid and add 4 cc of the oral solution to 120 cc of sterile I.V. water solution.

TREATMENT 2 - THEOPHYLLINE

Joseph Wybran and Andre Govaerts of Brussels, in an article published in Lancet, February 8, 1975, noted that there were reduced cancer deaths in asthmatics. They attributed this to the fact that asthmatics used theophylline for years. They reasoned that because theophylline stimulated the body to produce cyclic A.M.P., and cyclic A.M.P. causes cancer cells to revert to normal cells, this was the likely explanation.

Theophylline is very old and cannot be patented. So, as you might expect, Professor L.H. Opie (there's one in every bunch) commented in the October issue, that too much cyclic A.M.P. may be involved in causing irregular heart rhythms which could lead to a heart attack (so could his comment)! Thompson points out that two of the chemotherapeutic drugs used in cancer treatment are highly toxic to the heart and do cause heart attacks.

Professor Opie; what is too much A.M.P., how much theophylline can cause too much A.M.P., how many asthmatics die from theophylline causing heart attacks or is it from the stress on the heart (cor pulmonale) caused by the asthma? - Are you really serious?

****

SO GET WELL AND STAY WELL!

Robert EWilmer MD

295

LAST MINUTE IMPORTANT ADDITION

On the very last day of proof reading the manuscript for this book, I had a fortuitous introduction to Frederick Panker, the U.S. representative of Dr. Humberto Rangel of Mexico City. Dr. Rangel, who holds a specialists rank in Immunology, Infectious Disease and Pediatrics, has for fifteen years been treating patients with a autogenous vaccine obtained from a unique precipitate of the patients urine. Dr. Rangel has an impressive background which includes having been the Chief of Scientific Investigation for the Institute of Social Security for twelve years (1972-1984), Chief of Scientific Investigation in Mexico City and in the State of Michoacan.

Autogenous urine injections, as well as the drinking of ones own urine has been the subject of great controversy. I have also heard of vaccines being used but knew of no one who was doing it. Fred Panker showed me a batch of testimonials, most dealing with allergies, written and signed by the patients. One particular letter from the wife of a terminal pancreatic cancer patient touched me. ''... He only lived for another month but at least he was able to eat and enjoy his family and friends around him. And when his death finally came it was painless and very quick. I am glad .. I was able to give my husband a little bit more quality time.''

Later that day, Fred Panker faxed to me letters from Dr. Victor Manuel Espinoza Torres, the medical director of PETROLEOS MEXICANOS (The huge government-owned oil company) and Dr. Ovidio Pedraza Chanfreau, Past President of the Mexican Council of Pediatrics supporting Dr. Rangel's claims. I was impressed!

The list of ailments treated by the vaccine was extensive. I became interested when I saw cancer, multiple sclerosis, lupus, scleroderma, psoriasis and a host of other diseases where the usual treatments fail. What was especially interesting was the many emotional symptoms which responded to the therapy. It is not necessary to travel to Mexico for the vaccine. The treatment involves intradermal injections over an eight month period and costs $1,500.00. Improvement can usually be seen within 6 weeks and often immediately.

For further information contact:
Frederick Panker, Tel; 1-800-244-2088